The International Library

PSYCHOLOGICAL AND BIOLOGICAL FOUNDATIONS OF DREAM-INTERPRETATION

Founded by C. K. Ogden

The International Library of Psychology

GENERAL PSYCHOLOGY
In 38 Volumes

PSYCHOLOGICAL AND BIOLOGICAL FOUNDATIONS OF DREAM-INTERPRETATION

SAMUEL LOWY

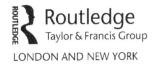

Routledge
Taylor & Francis Group

LONDON AND NEW YORK

First published in 1942 by
Routledge, Trench, Trubner & Co., Ltd.
2 Park Square, Milton Park, Abingdon, Oxfordshire OX14 4RN
711 Third Avenue, New York, NY 10017

First issued in paperback 2014

Routledge is an imprint of the Taylor and Francis Group, an informa business

British Library Cataloguing in Publication Data
A CIP catalogue record for this book
is available from the British Library

Psychological and Biological Foundations of Dream-Interpretation
ISBN 0415-21032-1
General Psychology: 38 Volumes
ISBN 0415-21129-8
The International Library of Psychology: 204 Volumes
ISBN 0415-19132-7

ISBN 13: 978-1-138-88249-2 (pbk)
ISBN 13: 978-0-415-21032-4 (hbk)

CONTENTS

FOREWORD

DR. SAMUEL LOWY is one of the most gifted of my pupils. His study of dream-interpretation does not pursue beaten trails, but breaks new ground, being the work of a pioneer. I am convinced that the book is of outstanding importance as a contribution to the study of the science of dreams. It contains the thoughts of an independent investigator, a man equipped with original ideas, endowed with a lively faculty for intuition, and enriched with abundant and ripe experience. Bearing in mind that Nietzsche wrote " A pupil who does not advance upon his teacher, does his teacher little credit ", I say frankly and unhesitatingly that Lowy has in this respect registered valuable and extensive improvements upon anything I have achieved. *Habent sua fata libelli*, but I am sure that if this book is ever published, it will be a lasting success, and will make a significant mark in the history of dream-interpretation. We are told that " talent originates in solitude, whereas character is formed amid the busy stream of life ". Now, this book manifests the author's talent for dream-interpretation, a talent that is inborn rather than acquired ; but it likewise shows the author's character, which is notable for independence.

It is my earnest hope that Lowy's Dream-Interpretation will enjoy the triumph it deserves.

DR. WILHELM STEKEL.

LONDON,
  13*th December*, 1938.

INTRODUCTION

ONE of the many tragedies arising out of the policy of hatred in recent years has been the enforced exile of innumerable men and women of science and learning from all parts of Europe. Those who were fortunate enough to escape with their lives have had to give up positions of security and dignity which enabled them to make their contributions to scientific knowledge freely and unhampered, and in foreign lands to accept (with gratitude) situations for the most part far below their attainments and records. What is so remarkable and so heartening is that many emigré scientists and doctors have continued to produce original work of merit in spite of all the difficulties that they have inevitably encountered. Dr. Samuel Lowy, the author of this book, belongs to the ranks of these undaunted workers. He was well on his way to establishing an excellent reputation as one of the younger generation of neuropsychiatrists working in Czechoslovakia, when his country was overrun by the enemy. In the country of his adoption he has managed to produce a work of considerable value and originality on dream-interpretation. There can be no final and definitive formulations of any aspects of human psychology, but any psychologist who seeks to review his subject against a general biological background deserves a respectful hearing ; for psychology is but biology seen in its non-material framework, and it is wise from time to time to shift the focus from one viewpoint to the other. I think that the readers of this book will find Dr. Lowy's psychobiological approach to the meaning and purpose of dreams unusually stimulating and satisfying. The author's well-reasoned views should appeal to the disciples of Freud, Jung and Adler, as well as to the more eclectic students of the psychology of dreams—in fact, the book should attract a wide circle of readers, both medical and non-medical. The *Psychological and Biological Foundations of Dream-Interpretation* is one of the most valuable contributions to that branch of psychology since Silberer's outstanding study of dreams published more than twenty years ago.

E. B. STRAUSS.

PREFACE

THE present small volume is intended as a psychological introduction to the science of dreams. An attempt is made in it to investigate, describe and give reasons for the various dream-mechanisms, so that their closer knowledge and understanding may give colour and justification to our psychotherapeutic dream-interpretations. I know from my own experience how much one would sometimes like to possess more secure knowledge of the foundations of dream-interpretation. Not everyone is able to sense and to grasp intuitively with his " psychological organ " the laws which are at work there ; although such a faculty of intuition is, in fact, one fundamental condition of our analytical work. Nevertheless, it will be useful to *know* what has been only *felt*, and to *understand* that which has been grasped by *intuition*. It is not possible here to give proofs and reasons as conclusive as is customary in other fields of science and research. What I have tried to do deserves rather the name of " approach ". Quite naturally, I deal with much that is well known and universally accepted, yet at the same time I present some conceptions which are new and different.

The basic views developed here are the result of my own research and of my own experience. The writings of most of the authors I quote in support of my theses, I was not acquainted with before the final revision of my manuscript.[1] (For ten years I lived in a comparatively small town, in Bratislava, the capital of Slovakia, where I had no modern psychoanalytic library at my disposal ; moreover, only recently have I learned to read English reasonably well.) Consequently, I must accept the sole responsibility for most of what I have written ; but it is possible that similar ideas have been expressed by other authors, perhaps in a different context. Such agreement between authors might even be regarded as supporting the probability of the ideas they hold in common. Of its kind this book is relatively novel both in its material and its manner of presentation, even where it deals with facts generally known. I think it will be found stimulating at least, and the desire of the author for critical

[1] This book is only an extract from a larger work.

xi

presentation and the greatest possible objectivity will—so I hope—be recognised. It is, of course, impossible in the science of dreams, and of psychoanalysis in general, to dispense altogether with theory and assumption, unless one is prepared to sacrifice to a too far-going cautiousness a wealth of ideas and possible resu'ts.

My large book on Special Dream-Interpretation cannot appear at the present time. A great part of the collected and systematised material is not at my disposal, due to existing conditions. I generally practise the so-called active psychoanalytical therapy, and I have in mind, above all, the needs of those who use this or a similar type of analytical treatment. The much too complimentary foreword by my teacher and fatherly friend, who died only recently in London, was written in fact for the complete larger work, whose general outline was familiar to him ; but primarily it refers to the various new views *here* expounded, whose early, embryonic form can be found in the various smaller articles which I wrote in my youth. This volume presents, however, a self-contained work, useful for the requirements of both the theorist and the practising psychotherapist.

S. L.

MANCHESTER,
    July, 1940.

MY deeply felt thanks are due to Professor J. C. Flugel who, in his unselfish way, and with the unbiased mind of a true scholar, read the original manuscript. It is a great honour for an author, unknown in this country, that this distinguished representative of British psychology, who was one of the earliest advocates of the psychoanalytical approach, should find the publication of his work worthwhile, even at a time so abounding in difficulties for the progress of higher science.

I am very grateful to Dr. D. S. Fairweather, M.A., M.D., M.R.C.P., D.P.M., Medical Officer of Rampton State Institute, and to Dr. T. Hart, Medical Officer of the County Mental Hospital, Prestwich, for their essential help in revising the English version of the book. They did this work with true interest in the topic, and not without personal friendship towards their colleague. They had frequently to face the " opinionated counter arguments " of the author, who often preferred an expression or a phrase, perhaps not quite usual, but which, according to his belief, was a better rendering of the intended thought.

I feel also indebted to Mr. Herbert Read, himself an author, familiar with modern psychological research, for his kindness in helping to prepare the book for the press.

I have also to thank Dr. E. B. Strauss, D.M., F.R.C.P., physician at St. Bartholomew's Hospital, for reviewing my book, and favouring me with the Introduction. I need not say how highly I value the interest shown to my work by this meritorious pioneer of modern psychiatry and medical psychology in Great Britain.

S. L.

February, 1942.

LIST OF A FEW FREQUENTLY USED
EXPRESSIONS

Affect-energy denotes the psycho-physiological energy, produced, and at work, under conditions which, in the subjective experience, are called emotional.

Affect-energetic nucleus denotes the formed nucleus of any circumscribed mental element, in its detachment from its conceptual component.

Conceptual dream-content is all that is " conceived " from the complex dream-experience, and which presents the material for the recollected and verbalised dream story. This expression was given preference over that of " images, ideas.", etc., because it is most apt to denote any kind of conceivable element. Besides, as the reader will see, we hold the opinion that all the dream-images represent ego-parts, and do not constitute true photographic pictures of perceptions.

Ego denotes, in this work, the whole psychosomatic personality, with its faculties of perceiving, feeling, conceiving and striving. The expression, therefore, covers only partly the meaning given to it in Freud's writings.

Subconscious (Scs.) designates any quality of a mental element beyond its character of being conscious. I do not feel justified in speaking of *unconscious*, apart from a very few, intended occasions, since we do not know enough about the sphere of total unconsciousness. Where we speak of the sphere of the unconscious, we have in mind the deepest layers, the " Id " of the Freudian terminology included.

Thinkable (and Unthinkable) denotes that quality of mental elements in virtue of which they are capable of being thought, i.e., to be shaped into circumscribed elements of conscious mental activity ; and respectively the reverse of it.

Waking thinking is used as an abbreviated expression for " the mode of thinking in waking state ". It is an expression which refers to the act, but not to the content of thinking.

Dream-image is the name we give to the result of the *dreaming-process*. When we speak simply of dreams, we mean the whole process of dreaming without wanting to distinguish these two separate aspects.

Anxiety-feeling corresponds to the German expression " Angst ". It denotes any morbid and unjustified fear, including states of fear for which there is no conscious reason.

CHAPTER I

THE DREAM AND ITS RELATION TO CONSCIOUS THOUGHT

(1) INTRODUCTION. It is my intention in this chapter to give a descriptive presentation of some details, pertaining to our subject and representing mainly the phenomenological aspect of it. I shall endeavour to do this in a critical fashion and in a constructive, logical order, showing the intrinsic mutual interrelations between the individual problems and trying at the same time, in a preliminary way at first, to throw some light on the background of the overt phenomena. Here, as throughout the book, particular attention will be paid to the needs of the younger therapist who wants to obtain a homogeneously unified view of the field of dreams, and who wants to know something about the justification for, and the foundation of, the interpretation of dreams. The discoveries and views of classical Freudian psychoanalysis will be amply considered in the further course of our investigations ; but they *do not* constitute the true framework for our discussions. *We* lay particular stress rather on the *manifest dream* ; it constitutes a safe guide for research, and undoubtedly the more certain and provable part of the study of the dream-problem can be carried out on it. However, both free associations and the interpreted, *latent dream-content* will also be included in the scope of the investigations. Biological aspects and physiological processes will also be discussed and stressed, in so far as they exert some influence on the dream-formation.

Our subject can be approached, partly by observing our own dreaming and our own dream-images, and partly by studying the great number of dreams, related to us by different people during their treatment, and analysed in the usual manner and to a degree attainable according to present-day knowledge.

Much has been written on this subject, both on individual and general problems. Much that has appeared in the literature is convincing and proven, or at least, interesting and well presented. It is natural that most of the authors have been members of the various contemporary psychological schools, and thus looked upon their work from *one* particular point of view.   The best book of this kind known to me is M. Nicoll's *Psychology of Dreams* (1920), which traces the ideas of Jung in an original manner.   Ratcliff's *The Nature of the Dreams* (1939) gives a brief but good survey on the different aspects and schools.   But no comparatively objective, " multi-dimensional " and creative compilation of the more generally accepted, because frequently confirmed, results has been attempted, to my knowledge, since the appearance of Sil-berer's book (1919).   I find it regrettable that this small volume has not been translated into English ; in its cautious method of enquiry and its endeavour to achieve scientific accuracy (as far as that can be reached in the field of psycho-logical research) it is definitely exemplary.   The present work, of course, is intended to mark a certain advance.   The bring-ing together of facts already known, the inferences drawn from time to time, and perhaps new formulations also, might be of interest to those who, because of the abundance of articles and books, treating of a wealth of observed facts, have not succeeded in forming a homogeneously unified impression of the subject.   For every scientifically trained mind the possess-ion of such a homogeneous foundation is an obvious necessity ; yet it also proves useful in the practical therapeutic work. I am too conscious of the only relative and limited value of my exposition ; also it was, unfortunately, necessary to omit from this publication much material derived from my own studies which I should like to have included.

(2) THE DREAMER AND HIS DREAM.   To the dreamer his dream is a vivid and relevant experience.   It represents an adventure, occurring while asleep, the more or less compli-cated actions of which seem of great interest to the dreamer, and are felt to concern him in some way or other.   This feeling accompanies even dream-events in whose course one's own person or concerns do not seem apparently to be in-volved ; there is always an emotionally coloured interest in the dream, even after awaking.   One has the feeling that the action of the dream took place in one's own sphere of interest. Sometimes we wake up with a feeling of pleasure, as if we had been enjoying tremendously our dreams of the night ; sometimes, and perhaps more frequently, there is an " after-feeling ", more or less well defined, of difficulty, of apprehen-sion, of struggle, of anxiety.   There seems to be an obvious

parallelism to the strongly affective way in which we react to the events of a play ; in both cases we may surmise that it is the process of *identification* which is responsible for this affective reverberation.

(3) THE MEMORY OF THE DREAM. There are frequently difficulties in the way of putting the events of the dream into words. They vary in degree and quality. Some parts of the dream, which we seemed to hold quite securely, mockingly elude our memory ; others can be revived by intense searching and concentration. Some remembered details arouse doubts as to their correct reproduction ; others again retain the character of obscurity and haziness (" The face was not clearly defined ; it was not possible to say who it was, though he was familiar to me ; it was some kind of object which I cannot describe, but in the dream I knew very well what it was for "). The recollection of the dream has always to surmount some resistance, some counter-pressure of varying intensity. It is, as if, between the dream and the act of remembering there were a long passage of time—or a different, strange world—diminishing the dream-reality. Or, as if, alternatively, some kind of psychic inhibition (" the censor " of Freud) put difficulties in the way of the memory.

This, surely, is a strange phenomenon ! Why do we possess at all a faculty for remembering our dreams in the waking state, if complete remembering is impeded in this way ? It seems almost as if dreams were really *not* destined for the knowledge of our waking consciousness. At all events, in the majority of the cases a dream is remembered only if there is a conative tendency to do so. This fact seems to constitute a certain argument against the view held by some that the dream is a finger-post for the waking life, a guide for the correct solution of the various problems of one's existence. However fitting and clever many of the examples may be, which are quoted in support of this view, the fact that dreams are usually forgotten speaks strongly against it. Dreams which appear to be of such " advising and warning " kind might be actually something different, something more. They contain not a mere plan for later life, not a counsel, nor a purely theoretical principle ; but they represent a self-contained, *concrete process* within the compass of the psyche. When, for instance, we refuse to see some real difficulty, some threatening complication, and exorcise it from our conscious thoughts, and then this reality appears in our dreams, this is probably not mere exhortation, or warning, but a sign that the subconscious psyche is usefully dealing with the difficulty in question, that it is mobilising and integrating the thought-processes relating thereto, that it is preparing itself for and against the eventuality, forming, as it were, " anti-bodies ", and *thus making up for what our conscious thinking neglected to do because it was unable to cope with it.* If, then, the real difficulty actually occurs, the psyche, the nervous system, the personality are not unprepared, not quite without mental " antitoxins ". It is, of course, better and more expedient when our waking consciousness takes note also of the problem, and aids in its solution. But the contribution of the dream, or of the deeper process it suggests, is a quite definite and self-contained reality ; it is no simple design of a plan, to be carried out, and still less mere idle phantasy.

I remember that during 1938, and in the first few months of 1939, I denied the possibility of a world war, both in my consciousness and in discussions with others. I could not bring myself to believe that my private life and scientific career, which, in spite of certain hopes and promise, had later met with difficulties at home because of the continuous political confusions in Europe, should even after my emigration, be cut short because of a world-shaking event of this kind. (In my mind, there was a different, gradual solution for all the wrong.) But in many of my dreams, I apparently foresaw the final catastrophe. Not the war itself, to be sure, but unfavourable conditions and the continuation of my struggle. For instance :

> 1. I am again at the beginning of my practice. My ignorance of English customs creates difficulties for me. I shall have to return home, but in my dream this " home " is like London. I see a soldier . . .[1]

Interpretation : What I lived through during the last few years at home, will now be continued in London. Indeed, I was less deeply moved and excited when war broke out than I had imagined earlier in my consciousness I would be. My psyche had to a certain degree anticipated the possible disappointment, without troubling my waking consciousness

---

[1] There is a certain advantage of citing one's own dreams, if one is concerned with the *sources* of the manifest dream-content, and not with the deeper interpretation, which latter would be likely to be " subjectively scotomised ".

(which would have been in this case even less expedient).
This function and method of working of the dream is the same
as when the dream fulfils a wish. *The wish-fulfilment in the
dream has its own value, its own satisfaction, without the necessity
of the dream being remembered.*[1] Eventual memory constitutes
a secondary gain.

The dream may be accessible to consciousness, at least
partly, but most decidedly it is not intended for the waking
consciousness. This view seems to be quite uncontestable.
If it were not so, the majority of dreams would not remain
unremembered. It is difficult to say that dreams carrying
significance, are more likely to be recollected. Also, the great
number of people—normal and neurotic alike—who seldom
become conscious of their dreams, would be put at a dis-
advantage, and quite unjustly. On the other hand, examples
like the one quoted above, show that dreams have a biological
function ; that they are not merely pictures, not only " psychic
formations ", but products of psychobiological significance.
This view will be developed in a later chapter.[2] Although,
as we have seen, the dream is not primarily destined for conscious memory, it is clear, on the other hand, that it is definitely
destined for being " consciously " experienced during sleep.
What the subconscious puts at the disposal of the dream-ego,
is meant to become " conscious " during dreaming. These
two different modes of becoming " conscious " ought not to
be confounded.[3]

(4) FORGETTING THE DREAM. Is forgetting of dreams a
genuine forgetting, similar in kind to that of a poem which we
knew well as children, and which we would readily recognise
as familiar on re-reading it ? Or is it rather a question merely
of feeling that we have forgotten something ; comparable
perhaps to the deceptive feeling of *déjà vu*, where one has the
impression of having lived previously through the present
moment ? It is sufficiently known that often in the course of
analysis the patient *does remember* fragments of dreams, or even
whole dreams, days after they have occurred, and he does so
with the distinct feeling of recollecting something once already
known, which was later forgotten. Freud considers this possibility the rule, and explains this behaviour as due to the

---

[1] Cf. Ch. VI (8) (9).
[2] The nature of this biological function is, in fact, more extensive than is explained in connection with the above dream. Cf. Ch. X.
[3] Cf. Ch. XII, p. 236.

removal in the meantime of some obstructing resistance. Everyone who himself carries out analyses, must acknowledge this beneficial effect of removal of inner inhibitions, because sometimes the analyst can evoke this effect *artificially* by means of an interpretation, explanation, or a suggestion. For instance, a man relates during his analysis a dream, the first half of which has remained firmly in his memory, but whose second half, which he dimly felt to have been more impressive and significant, has slipped his memory :

> **2a.** I see a dear friend of my youth ; she speaks to me. Then my sister passes us, looking older and rather sad. I feel sorry for her, but I go on cheerfully with my friend.

In the course of producing his free associations to this dream the patient mentions a particular weakness of this sister, her proneness to *vomiting*. Thereupon I ask him, if perhaps the forgotten part of the dream is connected with the topic of *disgust*, or *dislike*, or something similar. Suddenly he remembers having dreamed also about " large female genitals " full of mucus, which rather disgusted him ; somebody tried to swab them out, just as a doctor would. Further associations led to his dying father, to mucus in the throat of the sick man which tortured him and which had to be cleaned out ; then came still another part of the dream :

> **2b.** I see the genitals of my sister, and touch her gently.

Further associations helped to complete more fully the original dream, and to recognise the emotional background of it. The dreamer had promised his father to take care of his sister ; but his own complexes prevented him from doing so ; his love-affairs, his unstable reactions interfered with the duties life imposed upon him. Now his conscience stirs, he feels *guilty*, and cannot fully enjoy his love-life. He makes up for the neglect of his sister by intimacy in the world of his dreams. Yet this re-lived infantile sister-complex disturbs his libido in waking life. . . .

The following short dream was told by a young obsessional patient :

> **3.** I am travelling in the Tatra mountains,[1] with my friends.

---

[1] Czechoslovakia.

Associations : " I once thought of undertaking a long trip of this kind, so that I might escape, if only for a short time, from staying with my family, which to me is very burdensome." The boy found it very distressing to have his parents constantly quarrelling with each other, insulting each other, threatening to kill each other, but finally coming together sexually during the night. Unfortunately, the boy shared his parent's bedroom until his twenties, because his mother wished him to do so. I stated to him decisively that in his reveries, perhaps also in his forgotten night-dreams, he was constantly dealing with these facts and impressions. Then suddenly he remembered the following *dream of the previous day* :

> 4. I am on holiday, and put up at a cottage ; when I want to lie down, I notice under the bed two mad dogs fighting with each other.

The allusion to the above-mentioned pathogenic impressions and facts is clear enough.

In some other cases it has occurred to me that perhaps such dream-supplements *become capable of representation in consciousness and achieve the quality of being " thinkable " and " imaginable " only during the course of the analysis.* I had a patient who alleged that before undergoing treatment, he had never dreamt ; in the course of the treatment he remembered his dreams daily. Memories of his youth were few, all brought to the surface only through the analytical process. Instead of giving associations to his dreams, and instead of reproducing memories, he found it easier to complete his dreams, as originally related, by new details for half an hour or more. In his case the above-mentioned late maturation-process seems to be not an exceptional behaviour, but an intrinsic property of his reproductive capacity. On the other hand, one surely often notices how in the morning the dream-images could be reproduced in their full, logical sequence ; occasionally one even scribbles down notes about the dream ; but in the afternoon, when the hour for the treatment arrives, all this has disappeared, and even the notes may be incomprehensible. Sometimes during the transitional stage between sleep and awakening, one has the feeling that one has full knowledge of a complicated and intelligible coherent dream ; but on awakening one finds it quite impossible to seize even a fragment of it and to translate it into imagination and memory.

In such cases, I assume that the dream actually cannot be put into *word-expression* at all, or only under considerable difficulties, and with gaps ; i.e., it cannot be expressed in the modes and patterns of waking, conscious thinking. For several years I have suggested, and tried to propagate, the idea that the " deep " dream-event proper should be looked upon rather as a " non-conceptual, affect-energetic process ", while the conceptual forming into images, notions and ideas represents a second process.[1] So far, I have not noticed any response in the psychoanalytical literature ; though to me this conception seemed to offer a starting-point for some theoretical, and even practical, advance (disturbances of sleep ! Cf. Ch. X).[2] Not identical, although superficially similar, is the older assumption (Spitta) according to which everything remembered as a coherent text of the dream, is a product of the waking thought-system, a kind of secondary elaboration carried out by the logical thinking-mechanism ; only " in trying to reproduce the dream, we introduce order into the loosely connected elements of the dream-experience ".[3] But this assumption considers the conception, the thought-quality of the dream-elements as already completed, and deals only with their subsequent composition.   Besides, the subjective coherence of the dream experience *during dreaming* is a fact, which surely justifies the assumption just mentioned only to a very limited degree.   The essence and explanation of my theory shall follow now.

(5) THE NON-CONCEPTUAL, AFFECT-ENERGETIC DREAM-PROCESS.   Our ideas are not only thought, but also felt, experienced.   This affective component is the contribution of the " living ego " to the photographic image of the external impression, and constitutes in general a constant counterpart of the " lifeless " concept.   Every event, every experience, every representation of an external object and person, exerts a formative influence on the individual psychic life *only* in so far as it occasions in us " affects " of various qualities and

[1] The psychological terminology in this work is not always quite consistent with that of academic psychology ; inherent difficulties of the topic, and the individual aspect of the author, would have rendered unification, at present, impossible.   However, the understanding of the explanations will surely remain the chief aim of the reader ; and this would perhaps be made even more difficult by too strict adherence to the usual definitions of the expressions.

[2] Freud's theory on the infantile libidinous stimulus of dreaming, in fact, touches the present conception of the " affect-energetic, non-conceptual ", basic dream-process.

[3] Quoted by Freud.

quantities. Not the concepts and not the impressions of the external world in their objectivity, but the affective values, associated with and released by them, become functioning factors of our psyche. These affective counterparts of our concepts—the result of the complex ego-attitude to the external world and to all perceptions in general—make these external impressions properly *our very own*; they determine the exact disposition of concepts, images and ideas in us; these affective counterparts constitute the cement which binds the association-links together; they are responsible for both the quality and the intensity of the influence, exerted by individual psychic elements on the totality of our thinking and acting.[1]

The deepest dream-layers, perhaps the *scs.* beyond a certain depth in general, work with these affective constituents (I consider them as formed and circumscribed with regard to their content), and these affect-energetic dream-events stimulate in the " higher ", conceptual system adequate images which take their part in the final formation of the dream. The latter, then, is the conceptual image-expression of the deeper energetic events connected with the complexes. When, for instance, hostile sentiments are being worked off in the " deep " dream-process, images may appear in the projection on the conceptual level, dealing with hatred, war, etc. This is, of course, only schematically presented ; the process is surely more complicated. A dream of this kind, reported by a girl suffering from inhibited thinking and repugnance to life in general, ran like this :

> **5.** I am with some soldiers. Suddenly a man from the enemy camp appears and provokes a quarrel because of some marriage affair. I intervene and try to mediate and advise.

From these images we can conclude, with some degree of probability, that sentiments of a warlike, quarrelsome or provoking nature, and those having some bearing upon the problem of marriage, are at work in the psychic depths. Furthermore, we may assume the presence of respective energetic processes corresponding to the concepts of " meditation " and " giving advice ".[2]

---

[1] " Intuitive Dream-Interpretation in Psychotherapy." Lecture, 1930.
[2] " Peculiarities and Problems of Dreams during .Treatment." II., 1931.

Here is another dream by the same girl, conditioned by the same affects :

> **6.** My mother comes into the kitchen and begins an argument about some eggs which the hen has laid. I go away to have some peace and quiet.

Here also we find the motif of the quarrel, and the tendency towards reconciliation. We take the mother as representing an idea in the psyche of the girl ; she is prepared to leave, to forget this particular idea if harmony and peace require this.

This view of the deep dream-processes explains several peculiarities which differentiate the dream from waking thinking ; in particular, the superior affective content and experience quality of the dream-image, compared with its notion and cognitive content (Cf. Ch. V) ; and also that type of symbolical metamorphosis in which some scene which appears comparatively insignificant to conscious thinking, is coupled with a strong emotion, especially of anxiety (Cf. Ch. V (6), (7). (This is possible only because of the relatively loose connection between concept and affect-energetic component.) My theory also explains satisfactorily the rapid forgetting of dreams ; we are dealing here primarily not with a world of an essentially different content, but rather with a different category of thinking ; this qualitative difference must automatically render more difficult the transition of psychic elements from one level to the other. The position is similar in some ways to that of musical chords and melodies, which can be translated into word-expression, but only approximately ; however, the difference between the content of dream and waking thought is not quite so thorough ; it is rather *the quantitative proportion between affective and conceptual component of the mental elements, which differs, and which distinguishes the two categories of mental content.*

I should like here to discuss briefly the concept of " non-formulated thought " known in psychology, which seems to have some similarity and even relevance to our theme. We often have the feeling that we must search carefully and with a certain effort for the exactly correct expression of thoughts which, at first, are formulated only nebulously in our consciousness. We feel quite clearly that the formation proper of the thought, as content, has already been accomplished, but the mental struggle continues for the shaping of an expression of the thought (it is not the choice of the *correct* wording in sentences or phrases of the idea ; that process follows only later) ; the " feeling of the thought " (Apfelbach) is there, but not yet its verbal formulation in the so-called inner speech. This experience may help to make more intelligible my theory of the similar processes occurring in dreaming. But I should like to stress that in these " non-formulated thoughts " we are dealing with a thought-quality which is capable already of consciousness, a first step towards the fully formulated thought. (This is perhaps what Freud differentiates as *Sachvorstellung*, the concrete-idea, from the *Wortvorstellung*, the verbal-dea ; Cf. p. 13 below.) Yet what I ascribe to the deepest dream-process is rather some kind of affect-energy (perhaps this expression is not quite fitting, because " affect " usually denotes the *felt* reaction to an experience) ; some kind of formed and circumscribed psychic element which, however, is not provided yet with any " think-able " character. The analogy of electrically charged nuclei, i.e., electrons, may perhaps serve to make this conception more intelligible.

(6) If this separateness and relative independence of concept and effective nucleus were not a fact, it would be impossible for any symbolical transformation and substitution to take place, either in dreams or in the subconscious in general. The position would rather be, that each complete psychic element would consist of one definite concept and the affective counterpart, inseparably linked together. That this is not so, that affect-nucleus and concept *can* undergo changes dissociated from its counterpart, results in the motley variety of our dream world. I want to stress that the " affective nucleus " in the subconscious undergoes changes too, and that repression does not mean merely a formal " disguising " (Ch. II). The process of disguising, i.e., the replacement of the conceptual part by another conceptual element is, as a rule, an overt sign indicating the inner change of the nucleus in the *sbcs.*

The experienced analyst knows only too well how some psychic complex can be alluded to in the most diverse way. I once had a patient, in almost every one of whose dreams something *blue* occurred,—a blue ribbon, blue writing paper, or dress, a blue spot on the body, and so on. The solution was found later to lie in the " Bluebeard-complex ".   More frequently, one finds cases where some real, historical trauma is alluded to in the various dreams of the analytical period by means of different screen-images, and similarly, the persons who played a part in such pathogenic traumata are represented in various guises.   All this is so only because, as emphasised above, there is *no firm connection* between the psychic element in the *scs.* or in the dreaming level, and the concept pertaining to it.

It should be stressed that these hypothetical " affective elements " which take part in the dreaming-process, must not be mistaken for the dream-emotion, accompanying the experience as a whole.   (I have admitted that the expression " affect-nucleus " is misleading ; yet the physicist also speaks of the electric charge of a material as a whole, and in addition, of electrons as individual elements of their own.)   This dream-emotion, corresponding to the emotional reactions of waking life, is the total reaction of the ego to the total dream-event.   *Our* concept of the affect-nucleus, however, must be understood as an *isolated psychic element.*[1]

I believe that my conception of these subconscious psychic elements is complementary to Freud's views as developed in his *Das Unbewusste* (The Unconscious) written in 1915.   There he draws attention to the way in which in schizophrenic patients the *word-image* is obviously divorced from the *object-image* of the whole concept.   The various new and substitute formations of the schizophrene are caused more by similarity in expression than by similarity in kind and essence.—" There is little similarity of essence between the expression of a ' blackhead ' (comedo) and the ejaculation from the penis ; even less between the innumerable pores of the skin and the vagina ; but in the first case, we find that in both instances something gushes forth, and in the second case, we may remember the cynical saying : ' Opening is opening.'   It is the similarity of the verbal expression, not the similarity of the

---

[1] What Freud calls the " affective charge of an idea, of a content " is, as he indicates clearly, that part of the instinctive drive which belongs to the repressed thought, and which is either suppressed, or split off, or undergoes a qualitative change.   He, therefore, deals with the libidinous drive (and perhaps with the aggressive tendencies too) and not with what we have understood and described here, the affect-nucleus of each particular concept, each individual idea.   Of course, the individual elements which pertain to an elaborate libidinous wish, approximate, and are closely related to, the affective charge conceived as the totality of the drive.   *But here we have not in mind mere instinctively conditioned compound complexes.*

essence of the things which (in one particular case) has pre-scribed the substitution." We have to admit, of course, that there exists a certain similarity of form behind the expressive identity ; what Freud wants to point out is the lack of " essen-tial similarity ". The schizophrene, as is well known, uses these substitute images as natural parts of his conscious thought, since he has lost the proper concepts. Freud con-cludes from this that, in principle, an idea consists of two distinct components, the " concrete idea " (*Sachvorstellung*) and the " verbal idea " (*Wortvorstellung*). " The conscious idea embraces the concrete idea plus the appropriate word idea ; the unconscious idea [1] consists solely of the concrete idea. In the process of repression, the repressed idea content is denied super-cathexis by the verbal component. The idea which in this way is being verbally unrepresented remains in the unconscious as a repressed mental element."

However, one does justice to the facts only if one attributes an affective nucleus to the total concept. Only a non-conceptual element is capable of such deep-seated trans-formations as we meet with, particularly in dreams ; no conceptual representation alone can explain how in a series of dreams one particular, symbolised person, is represented by a large number of other persons. Verbal idea, concrete idea, and the basic affect-nucleus attached to the latter, which constitutes the " life " and the felt quality of the psychic elements, are then the schematically distinct components of each idea, of each psychic element in general. Verbal and concrete ideas already imply conceptual thought-quality. *The deepest dream-process, however, works with non-conceptual elements. The experienced dream-image, perceived while sleeping, already con-tains the conceptual concrete idea. The dream which is represented in waking thought, i.e., which is remembered, has in addition the verbal idea.*

I think it is justified to put forward such hypotheses, if one can thus explain the variety of events more clearly. The verbal idea (not the word-expression as word-sound), of course, circumscribes and limits the element entirely ; the subconscious root, the concrete idea, is connected with associa-tions pertaining still to the core of the notion ; but it is the detached affect-nucleus which undergoes far-reaching changes through various loose associative processes.

[1] That probably means : after having become unconscious through repression.

(7) If then the dreaming-process has dealt with elements or combinations of elements which by their very nature are largely incapable of being put into words, it is easy to see how one can have a vivid feeling of having dreamt a good deal, but at the same time be quite unable to recollect anything. Such a feeling, such a subjective impression, arises from the non-conceptual process of the dream-experience, and has no bearing on any true conceptual content, as it is understood in the sphere of conscious thinking, knowing and forgetting. Even when a dream *is* remembered to a degree complete for the subjective feeling, we may take it for granted that there is a disproportion of size between the extent of the original depth-process and that part which has become conscious. It is generally acknowledged that the processes of the unconscious and subconscious exceed those of the conscious sphere. I would say that there is a similarity to that quantitative difference existing between our limited self-perceptive knowledge of our bodily processes and the inconceivable wealth of the factual events. There is every reason to assume that this difference in extensity implies also one in quality. Many constant complexes of the *scs.* are very probably quite incapable of being thought of; they do not pertain to the world of causal and logical categories, but to that of the elementary life-instincts. In Freud's opinion, as is known, the unconscious is altogether void of regard for time and real possibility. Our idea of " unthinkable " subconscious contents is a supplement to his conception.

True, we can imagine and conceive a good deal of the sphere of the self-preserving drives, as far as they lead to the feeling of hunger and thirst, etc., just because these instincts *have* to result in some overt form of purposive action. Similarly, we are able to conceive concretely much from perhaps even the broader sphere of sexuality and the finer libidinous processes. But all the side-branches and wide ramifications of the instinctive processes, occurring deeply inside the organism, inside the personality and all their intermediate stages and effects—surely though they reach the deepest unconscious, the Id, and enter from there also the dream-consciousness—yet they remain far indeed from the sphere of waking thought and " thinkability " in the usual sense.

Capacity for becoming " thinkable " is, of course, not identical with that of becoming " conscious ". An infantile

Œdipus-complex is surely " capable of being thought of ",
but as a rule not capable of remaining fully conscious, particularly when its undesirable strength disturbs the mental
development, and life harmony in general. *We must then
regard the a priori incapacity of dream elements for becoming " thinkable " as one important factor, responsible for the forgetting of dreams,
or for making the recollection difficult and only insufficient.* It is
quite likely that frequently even those parts of the dream
which are capable of being thought, are becoming lost to
reproductive memory because of their close connection with
elements " not capable of being thought ". They are being
pushed back into forgetfulness. This is probably the situation
when the dreamer can remember only one word, one single
fragment, as the sole remnant of a longer dream, and when
he is also unable to produce any free associations. I am, of
course, aware that such phenomena occur frequently during
the period of " resistance " in the analysis ; and apart from
this, we have accepted the fact that dreams which were
once conscious, *may* be subsequently forgotten. Yet, I consider it highly probable that *in such difficult periods of treatment,
a great deal of dreaming occurs actually in the imperfect, non-conceptual
manner above described* ; first, because of the emotional " resistance " ; secondly, because the contents which are being
" worked-up " and shaped by the analytical process, have not
yet crystalised out sufficiently to be capable of being formed
in thought quality (" thinkable ") ; further, because the psychoenergetic processes occurring in the deep layers at that
particular stage of analysis, have not yet succeeded in gaining
contact with some of the repressed material which *was* originally capable of being thought and of becoming conscious.

These few remarks may serve as a contribution to the
doctrine of the " analytic resistance ". To my mind, the
phenomenon of resistance is always only partly a sign of
repression in the sense of " inability for becoming conscious " ;
largely it is a question of immaturity or incapability for
" becoming thinkable " at all ; a quality, assumed by a large
part of pathological complexes during their repression.
Furthermore, I have already hinted at the supposed fact,
which I shall explain at greater length in the chapter on
symbolism, that *all* elements of consciousness undergo a
more or less essential transformation in their subconscious
counterpart.

(8) When I maintained earlier that some dream-supplements became capable of being thought, only in the course
of the following day, or during the analytical hour, and that
their transformation and shaping were completed only when
they were actually remembered, I meant to imply that *one*
possible reason for the obstruction of the dream-recollection
lay in the *yet uncompleted development* of the dream-material
into a form capable of being thought and put into word-
expression.   For a number of cases, Freud assumed that the
dream-work proper lasted through many hours, and that its
working was subjectively " felt " all the time ;   though the
resulting dream-image was, in fact, . the only remaining
product.   (*Interp. of Dreams*, Ch. VII.)   It is better—and we
are reaching a more unified, homogeneous conception—if we
assume here too, that that part of the " dream " which is not
remembered, was experienced only in an affect-energetic
quality, which would not permit of its becoming " thinkable "
and this resulted in the feeling of forgetting.

We see that in considering the view here propounded,
there appears a close relation between the process of dreaming
on the one hand, and the process of analysis on the other.
After all, analysis implies largely reduction or restoration of
subconscious (and perhaps *un*conscious) contents to conscious
and thinkable material ;   here we are primarily interested in
the latter quality.   The very same tendency reveals itself in
the process of verbalisation which accompanies the remembering of the dream, and even in the previous association of the
deeper affect-energetic process with the " conceptual image-
layer " during the dreaming-experience.   In this connection,
we may remember that frequently individuals who dream
little in the ordinary way, begin to dream more, and even
much, in the course of a satisfactory analysis.   This observation has in general been explained only by the greater attention
which the patients give to their dreaming in an endeavour
to remember them.   I firmly believe that this interesting
phenomenon, which is amazing to the patient too, has *dynamic*
causes.   The analytical process facilitates the formation of
more *thinkable material*, and this results in the increasing production of dreams, which are capable of being thought and
remembered.

(9) In this connection we may also discuss the question of
" sound, dreamless sleep ".   Freud speaks of a sleep, free

from irritation and stimulation, in line with his view that the dream is a kind of *guardian of sleep*, and that all irritating stimuli, arising during sleep, are being side-tracked through the hallucinatory experience of the dream. But the forgetting of dreams in certain stages of analysis, which latter we definitely recognise in many ways, e.g., by the behaviour of the patient, as periods of " resistance ", and which must be admitted to be due to deeper, inner difficulties, raises a doubt in our minds about his explanation (particularly if this forgetting occurs in patients who previously dreamed frequently) ; so, too, does the poverty of dreams of many border-line psychotic individuals. I should suggest the following formula to cover all cases : Dreamlessness is always caused by non-conceptual dreaming (we leave out of consideration here the cases of actual forgetting). It is brought about by factually sound sleep in one group of individuals (dreams of the deepest sleep levels are probably altogether non-conceptual [1]) ; while in other cases, viz., those of unhealthy psychic structures, it is caused by a greater incapacity of their mental content for becoming conscious, or even more, for being " capable of being thought " at all. In the dreamless periods of analysis, the causation is similar.

I can only repeat that everything we know about the way in which the *scs.* layer works, makes it very likely that conscious contents displaced there, undergo a continuous change, which most likely lies in the direction of the " non-conceptual ". I believe also that an experience which cannot be assimilated satisfactorily, will have to suffer more and more this process of " de-conceptualisation ".

(10) It is well known that some dreams remain in memory for decades, in all their vividness and completeness. As detailed analyses have shown, the deeper content of such dreams cover motifs, important and characteristic of the person in question, and are, therefore, supported and strengthened by a large number of associations which enable them to resist the normal course of forgetting. We know that it is very instructive to enquire after the earliest conscious memory of the individual. Be the scene remembered ever so small and apparently unimportant, it is characteristic of a

---

[1] De Sanctis maintains : " It is quite probable that the dreams of very deep sleep—supposing the dreamer could reproduce them—would be expressible in a different form only (manifest content) ; or more likely, they would not be expressible at all." To my mind, the latter possibility is the only correct one.

certain attitude and aspect of the individual's personality. From the multiplicity of impressions this *one* particular scene has been electively retained as a frame, a receptacle, a short-hand expression of a complicated content.[1] The sense, the significance of this small episode lies in its background, its associations, its symbolic content. Dream-memories outlasting the years, should be regarded in a similar manner. One might query the purpose, the teleological significance of these memories ; for, as we have explained above, conscious memory, as such, does not seem to form part of the intrinsic purpose of dreaming. In another context, I shall quote a passage from Bjerre,[2] in which he maintains that subconscious elements appear from time to time in dreams, in order that they may not become quite immobile, quite unconscious, and thus incapable of being reproduced, should the psychological necessity for such reproduction arise. It really seems to be a necessity for the psychic organisation to keep open certain associative channels between conscious and deeper levels. It is hardly possible for me to say more about these phenomena.

(II) THE STRANGENESS OF DREAMS. The dream-content appears more or less strange to waking consciousness ; sometimes only in its details, mostly, however, in its totality. The dream is a message from a different ego-world. Frequently, there is only the feeling of surprise. I dreamed the other day that " I am walking arm-in-arm with a girl from my birthplace, and we are having an animated conversation ". Now, I had not seen this girl for over 20 years ; furthermore, she has been dead for 10 years. It is true that I was fond of her—she was my colleague at school and later my pupil ; also she thought highly of my abilities, and this, naturally, used to flatter my vanity. But in reality our relationship was never as close as it appeared in the dream. Admittedly, in the days preceding the dream I had thought of her with a certain affection.

Now the dream appeared to me not only agreeable, but also quite natural, self-evident even after awakening. It seems probable that others too experience such " improbable " dreams which have no trace of strangeness ; one can only be sure of this fact in one's own case. I should like to say in this connection that it is not the degree of coincidence with reality or close possibility which decides the amount of strange-

---

[1] See on " screen-memories ", Ch. IV, p. 104.   [2] Ch. XII, p. 201.

ness felt. Even though the dream, just quoted, had certain relations to the real events, to the long past, and to recent remembering, both its particular mode of action and its *coefficient of reality* have a very low degree of probability, both with regard to their real historical background, as mentioned, and even less for the present, because she died years ago. (I am not taking into account the deeper psychoanalytic interpretation, but only the manifest dream as it appeared originally. Incidentally, I want to stress the fact that *the manifest dream has always its own significance* [1]; at least as a means of a connecting function. Cf. Ch. XII, p. 201–2.) The feeling of strangeness depends exclusively on the kind of relation obtaining between *dream-content* (manifest and latent together) and the *conscious tendencies of the ego*. Many other dreams, which are perhaps nearer to historical reality and possibility, arouse the impression of strangeness, if they *do not* fulfil positively this condition. Thus I dreamed that " one of my brothers would soon enter the Civil Service ". There is nothing factual in this dream either. Nevertheless, the evening before I had been considering the advantages of a secure post in these uncertain, revolutionary times. (On the beneficial function of such a displacement. Cf. Ch. II.) Such a dependent position, however, would arouse in me personally a sense of too great limitation, so that the thought of it strikes me as strange and disagreeable even in connection with my brother. As a matter of fact, he *is* employed in business, i.e., tied down and having a fixed salary, conditions similar to those of the Civil Service. For him, therefore, employment by the State would constitute even a certain advantage, because it would mean at the same time more security for his immediate future. But, as I said, the thought of such a position, *in association with myself*, is so unnatural to me that the whole dream appeared very strange. We are dealing then, with a factor connected closely with one's own personal sentimental attitude towards the deeper dream content ; not with the logical intelligibility or incomprehensibility of the manifest dream. I should, therefore, suggest that the dreamer be questioned about these accompanying feelings of strangeness or familiarity ; his answer may contain certain, valuable hints for the therapist-interpreter.

(12) Least difficulty in establishing contact with waking

[1] Cf. also V (9) and XII (4), p. 196.

thought and understanding is encountered in those dreams which deal with wishes and fears of the conscious field ; also those which represent physiological needs occurring during sleep. The feeling of strangeness is related, from the purely descriptive viewpoint, to various categories of the world of ideas : strange or partly changed faces ; unknown or modified localities ; actions of persons known to us, which in the given connection are unthinkable, unusual, very surprising, or even shocking ; also our own rôle in the dream-event when it is contrary to our views, conscious intentions, or actual advantages ; neglect of æsthetic considerations and of tact ; the non-existence of social and moral barriers, of financial and even physical limitations. A few interesting examples may follow :

> **7.** The dreamer smokes a cigar ; at first it does not burn well. Then he pulls it over his head, like a cap.

This happened in the dream as a matter of course. The cigar in the place of a cap *did not* create any impression of the unusual, until after awakening ; the only complaint during dreaming was that it was rather difficult to put the cap on because it was too narrow. The dreamer suffered from an exceptionally grave form of neurosis ; impotency, compulsion of masturbation and subsequent suicidal impulses, once actually attempted ; the background consisted of masturbation-phantasies of child murder, preceded by rape. The interpretation of the dream-content might be put into the following words : This sexual conflict, which has led to impotency (the badly burning cigar) " burned his conscience " (head). Also, the patient's subconscious interest started to be directed towards his hidden pathological thoughts (brain), rather than towards the overt symptom of the malfunctioning genital. (The treatment of this difficult case ended with considerable success.[1])

Here is another dream, which I did not analyse :

> **8.** The dreamer had pointed leaves instead of finger-nails, and was working rhythmically with her hands ; in the dream this did not seem at all unusual or unreal.

---

[1] In commenting on the good or indifferent results attained in some difficult cases, we want only to contribute to the case-material of the psychological literature, in view of the, at times, considerable number of disappointing limitations one encounters in the course of practical work.

I myself once dreamed :

> 9. Psychiatric lecture, or scientific meeting. On my left, I see the professor reading from a book in his usual *boring* manner. On my right there is a *woman*. I fetch a piece of cake from the table, although I am not at all hungry, and eat it. Then suddenly it is like a banquet, but at the same time, the lecture continues. My neighbour on the right takes a sweet which *I had not noticed* earlier and eats it. I have the feeling the sugar in the sweet may taste good, but it would surely be bad for gastritis. I awake with a feeling of indigestion.

To explain the superficial aspects of this dream, it may be pointed out that pure psychiatry, because of its comparative therapeutic limitations, often appeared a trifle irksome to me, and I frequently thought it would be a suitable field for industrious and kind women ; I knew several female assistants who did very well in this work. I myself have never delved deeply into the theory of the subject, in so far as it went beyond the important practical aspects, and I found the lectures amusing rather than of real importance (I admit this was a too subjective impression). My psychiatric self, therefore, appears in the dream as a *woman*, thus underestimating this profession. (She, however, finds something which I failed to see ? Envy ? For several years now the " scientific affection " of the author belongs to neurology ; it seems to offer more to his special way of doing psychology.)

For some time, I used to write down my dreams in order to check the results of my dream-investigations by material from my own dreams ; in this way I found that my dreams are relatively lacking in apparently " non-logical " elements ; that, in other words, my dreams are influenced very strongly by the need for logical order, which I think is fairly marked in my waking thinking. The problem of the various types of dreamers [1] have not yet been dealt with in a proper and systematic way by psychologists. [2] In the chapter on the World of Dreaming, we will take up again the phenomenon of illogical motifs.

Heraclitus, who lived in the fourth century B.C., had already maintained that *dreams have a reality of their own*. Fechner,

---

[1] Cf. Ch. XII (21) ; Cf. also p. 108.
[2] Pierce's *Dreams and Personality*, 1931 (a good start to this task), did not come to my notice until this manuscript was finished.

who is quoted by Freud, comes to the conclusion that the
" arena of the dream " is not identical with that of waking
life. " Neither the simple depression of conscious life under
the main threshold, nor the distraction of the attention from
the influences of the other world suffices to explain the peculiarities of dream life as compared with waking life. If the
arena of psychophysical activity were the same during the
sleeping and the waking state, the dream could only be a
continuation of the waking ideational life at a lower degree
of intensity, so that it would have to partake of the forms and
material of the latter. But this is by no means the case."
Because with regard to, and towards, external reality normal
human beings are almost similar—they have to be so for the
sake of social life—we may expect their deeper constitutional
differences to become all the more marked and apparent in
their dreams.

(13) The unreal and impossible quality of the dream-
events is usually *not* experienced, not recognised as such
during the dreaming-process ; if it is, we are dealing with
an encroachment by waking criticism. Freud maintains that
the formative processes of the dream do *not* produce any
genuine judgments, causal or logical arguments, or speeches ;
all these elements are borrowed from waking thought. We
do not follow this, for him, fundamental differentiation ; for
our modern technique of interpretation *everything is dream
which has become part of the dream-image.* Freud's distinction
seems to follow from his whole conception of dreams and
dreaming. (Cf. Ch. VI.) It is, however, often possible to
confirm his thesis that everything that is said in the dream
is merely reproduction ; a few cases gave me the opportunity
of finding this. The lack of success in discovering the historical sources is, of course, *no* cogent counterproof ; surely,
one may take the word of an analyst of such experience as
Freud, who carried out many and *long lasting* analyses, and
thus had ample opportunities for tracing the historical background of the various dream elements. On the other hand,
I must stress the point that according to my own experiences
the position of a sentence in the newly formed dream often
imparts to it a *different significance* and content.[1] This is true
to an even greater extent in the case of judgments in dream.
Let me quote a dream from Stekel's *The Language of the Dream,*

[1] Compare a similar fact with regard to associations. Ch. IV (1).

Ch. XIII. I believe it furnishes a good illustration of the point mentioned :

> **10.** Mary offers me her *scarf-pin* as a present. I refuse it, saying, " I thank you, but you know that pins as presents bring *misfortune*. Also, I shall make you a present of another, better (warmer, more alive) pin."

Mary is the dreamer's fiancée, and brought to his sister some presents ; but she retained her beautiful *scarf-pin*. The dreamer wanted her to give this brooch, too, to his sister Rose. Mary answered : " I can't do that. You know that pins as presents bring *misfortune*." It is easy to see how the historical sentence reappears in the dream in a changed fashion, being spoken by the dreamer and being completed by additional words. Stekel goes on to quote an interesting remark of Freud's : " One finds that it is the dream which at times gives the correct text of the *compulsive command*, of which in the waking consciousness of the patient, only a fragmentary and distorted form is present ; these full commands appear in the dreams as *speeches*, contrary to the rule, that speeches in the dream are simply reproductions of speeches made by somebody during the day."

The dreamer was suffering from a grave conflict, which had the formula : fiancée or sister. The dream betrays his compulsive idea : he wants Mary to renounce the pin (genitals). The friendly sentence, so Stekel explains, is really directed towards the sister : " Although you have not received the scarf-pin of my bride, you have something more valuable, namely, my deep love." When he informed his sister about his intention to marry, she threatened to take a lover herself. This threat excited and annoyed him a good deal. " That would be a great *misfortune* for me." (See the corresponding expression in the dream.) Those acquainted with the world of dreams and neuroses, will not be astonished that the dream changes quoted words and that consequently the interpreter, on his side, has to carry out similar, but reverse changes. The words, in the dream addressed to his fiancée, are really meant for the sister. Without splitting up the speech in this manner, and relating at least the second part to the sister, it is difficult to see any coherent content in the dream.

(14) THE MEANINGFULNESS OF THE DREAM. The fact that dreams are in principle meaningful is shown, in my opinion, by

those dream-images which appear quite intelligible, without additional analysis, even if they do not reproduce facts of reality. I do not refer here to simple day-residues (Freud), i.e., mere photographic reproductions of events and thoughts of waking life. Such reproduction itself can hardly be looked upon as creative and meaningful. I mean, rather, dreams which show a certain clear continuity with waking life ; dreams in which wishes, tendencies and apprehensions of conscious life *are continued* in some logical form. If then it is established that a relatively small, but constant, percentage of dreams does possess a sensible content, a " meaning ", independent from any artificial process of interpretation, we should assume it in principle for all the dreams. Phenomena of nature in general, and the physiological functions of living beings in particular, reveal a certain constancy, regularity and uniformity ; they are (if we except pathological conditions) not now regular and now irregular. Waking thoughts, too, are always meaningful ; if not always objectively, with regard to reality and expediency, they are, subjectively at least, sensible and meaningful. Thinking, I should define as the subjective way of regarding both the external and internal world, i.e., considering them in their totality and continuously, from the viewpoint of one's own social position and safety, one's own aims, desires and fears. Adler says that the most important task of thinking is anticipating action and events. (The Nervous Constitution, Ch. III.)

We find sense in the apparently incomprehensible dream-images, i.e., we discover a bridge between the dream-world and the thought-world of waking life, only when we are prepared to regard the dream or some of its parts, as *symbolic disguises of a quite different content*,[1] as a condensed formation which is capable of extension and indeed *in need* of completion.

If we ask, why some dreams or parts of dreams are intelligible directly to our waking thought, while others make sense only after more or less extensive analytical elaboration, we can give only *one* objectively acceptable answer. The two kinds of dream-contents point to a mixture between two different types of formation process, one may call them also two different systems, which are at work at the time of shaping of the respective dream-image. The fact that this mixture occurs,

[1] Cf. Ch. II.

and the degree in which the two systems participate, seem to have no importance for the meaning of the dream ; they are more a secondary consequence than something essential, i.e., mere consequence of the accidental ratio in the composition of the dream-consciousness at a given moment.[1]

When a certain dream fragment, perhaps quite intelligible and logical in itself, does not fit in well with the rest of the dream-content, we also usually try to de-symbolise and to decipher it. Quite frequently, it is possible later to gain the conviction that this procedure and conjecture was well justified. It must, however, be said in all honesty : *dream interpretation is always a process of groping and feeling one's way, a subjective manner of treating the dream material.* What seems established in the science of dream interpretation, is the knowledge of certain rules, by whose help one is enabled to draw conclusions with regard to conscious thought-elements, or those capable of becoming conscious, from the, at first, quite unintelligible material of the dream. Interpretation, then, is fundamentally an attempt to reduce the dream-content to conscious and intelligible thought. But as long as no proof was possible, it could not but remain questionable, whether in any particular case we were justified in assuming some kind of symbolical expression behind a particular part of the dream, or whether we are dealing with a disguise effected by distortion, substitution, or with some allusion to an intention through presentation of the contrary, or through transposition ; whether we were correct in looking upon some part of the dream as the deposit of historical events, or as representation of " functional " psychic attitudes ; in brief, whether the application of any particular mode of interpretation was warranted in a given case. In the chapter on Symbolism, we shall deal at greater length with the problem of dream-formation ; and in the chapter on Interpretation also these problems will be dealt with more concretely.

Everything that is later confirmed by information given by the dreamer, naturally proves itself to be a correct supposition. Every interpretation, too, which upon communication to the patient aids the progress of analysis, through removal of inhibitions or resistances to the treatment, seems at least justified, and to a certain extent probably correct. In several cases, it can be shown and even definitely proved, that one

[1] Cf. Ch. II (2), (10).

particular element of the dream is connected with a very large number of thought-elements, and also that the wording of the dream might be understood both in its literal, manifest form and in its symbolic meaning. The most obvious proof of condensation is presented by the mixing up of several localities in the dream, in the compound-formation of many dream-figures, and lastly, in the obvious association of two or more associative elements with *one* dream-element. But it will never be possible to reduce the dream-elements completely to conscious thoughts; the reason, as pointed out above, being that there is a quantitative and qualitative incongruity between the two psychic spheres. What, therefore, has been regarded above as the main reason for the manifold difficulties in recollecting dreams is, of course, at the same time, and to an even greater degree, the source of our difficulties in interpretation. Long, complicated dreams, with many embellishing details will serve in particular as proof for the existence of this disproportion. In the case of such dreams, we must remain content with an intelligible interpretation of the main theme of the " story "[1]; at times we are even reduced to the extraction of a single element from the total dream, without a possibility of giving even approximate explanation of the remaining details. Admittedly, more of these details become more intelligible through free associations. With regard to the majority, however, we must assume that although they *all* give expression to some *scs.* element, and they all are necessary in order to represent the whole complicated state of affairs in the depths of the psyche, yet the " totality " of these affairs in the *scs.* and *ucs.* remain for us only incompletely capable of being consciously thought. For all practical purposes, therefore, we must rest content in being able to utilise only certain elements. It is fortunate indeed that for therapeutic purposes such a procedure is quite sufficient. The fact that it is possible, of course, to obtain innumerable associations in response to each element of the dream, proves only the extent of the ramification of psychic elements; not their actually close relation to the meaning of the dream. A large number of these associations belong to the individual element as considered separately, but not to the dream-meaning, not to *that* content which this element has in constituting a part of the homogeneous

[1] Simplification of the dream (Stekel).

total dream. The figure of the *father*, for instance, may stand surely *also* for the idea of paternity, or for the husband of the mother, or for a special human quality represented by that father-individual. Not always do all possible meanings belong to the dream-totality. The nature of free associations will be dealt with at greater length in Ch. IV.

CHAPTER II

INTRODUCTION TO DREAM SYMBOLISM

(1) IT is a well-established fact that elements of waking thought and also subconscious contents both reappear in the dream-image under symbolic disguises. Most dreams can be brought into relation with the individual world of the dreamer's conscious, and with the ways of logical-realistic thinking in general, *only* if certain elements of the dream are deciphered and interpreted, by not taking the manifest form literally and by considering it as a mere substitute-formation. This symbolic transformation of the dream embraces partly the individual elements of the whole scene, and partly the fundamental action itself. One finds frequently that in some dreams the basic action, at least, is depicted in keeping with the usual modes of waking thought, and that only a few details appear so unreal, i.e., so impossible and unintelligible, that they require interpretation—a reduction to a different meaning—before they can be fitted intelligibly into their context. Such is the dream of a man who used to reproach his fiancée at times for certain small insincerities :

> **11.** I have to go through a very narrow passage, which I can manage only with difficulties, crawling on my stomach. When I reach the kitchen I meet B's mother and ask for her daughter. I assume the girl is asleep in the next room. But her mother tells me that B will not be home till five, that she has been going out to work since September. I shout in great anger : " Why did she keep that secret from me ? She is always full of lies, of insincerity ; I am hurt . . ."

There is no trace of any photographic reproduction, of anything factual, historically correct, in this dream, apart from the fact that little squabbles with regard to sincerity had actually taken place a few times. Not even the locality of the dream-event corresponds in the least with the actual place in question. (Associations to which we shall pay no attention in this connection, led back to the third year of the dreamer's life ; but even this only in passing.) In spite of all this, the action itself is quite possible in reality ; it is even quite readily intelligible as a continuation and elaboration of the conscious theme : " She is not sincere enough." Only one part of the dream, that dealing with the dreamer's crawling through the narrow passage, is quite alien to reality and to the possibilities of waking life ; no kitchen entrance is constructed in this fashion, and certainly this is not the proper way for a friend of the family, for the fiancé of the daughter of the house, to enter. Consequently, it seemed reasonable to regard this element as unreal, non-genuine, in its manifest form, i.e., symbolic. In view of the known facts, it was easy to see in this dream-element an allusion to the difficulties which stood in the way of this marriage.

(2) One meets quite frequently with such " mixed " dreams, in whose construction two different forming systems take part ; where it is obvious that the dream level is in connection *both* with the system of conscious thought and that of symbolical expression and this at the same time. I think we are justified in concluding that though the level at which the dream originates, is the subconscious—after all sleep implies the state of not being conscious—nevertheless this dream-subconscious is not to be localised in the deepest instinctive level of the psyche, designated by Freud as the Id.[1] In general, sleep does not seem to imply complete regression to the Id, only an approximation to this condition, through extensive, but incomplete, turning away from the reality of the outer world. (A mother, worried about her small or sick child, may sleep quite soundly in spite of loud noises from the environment, but she will wake up immediately the beloved child cries or moans ever so softly.) I want to imply, also, that *symbol formation itself* does not belong to these deep levels. The close relation of dream symbolism to the symbolism of art and language would itself argue against such an assumption. It is true, the impulse (and the capacity) to employ this mode of expression comes, even in the conscious state, from the deeper, affective psychic levels, from a subconscious sphere, near to the world of pure " feelings " ; definitely not from " thinking " which is orientated towards clarity and precision ; under no conditions, however, does it emerge from the deepest Id. (The patterns of such symbols, however, constitute one special part of our innate mental dispositions.) *Symbolic expression implies some kind of " creating " and shaping.* De Sanctis similarly maintained that " it is improbable that dream symbols should originate rather from the depths of the Unconscious

[1] Cf. XII (16), p. 230.

(inherited, racial, mythical, infantile) than from waking consciousness ".

(3) The whole problem of dreaming, the question of how and where the dream formation takes place, put considerable difficulties in the way of objective research in virtue of the peculiarities of the material which constitutes the subject of the investigation ; speculation and hypothesis naturally play a large part in even the most cautious exposition. Yet it is the dream symbolism more than any other part of this field, which places the greatest obstacles in the way of systematic description, exposition and proof. In spite of the comparatively large amount of results which have been collected, the gaps in our knowledge seem too great, and the unanswered questions too many, to make easy a clear, coherent exposition of this particular problem, and to enable us to link together into a homogeneous unity the individual findings. It is certain that the interpretation given in several cases, can be regarded as approximately correct and even proven ; equally certain is the existence of several established symbolic equations. However, the field where our knowing and even our imagining does not extend, is yet larger than our positive knowledge, and accordingly it is difficult at present to build up a satisfactory doctrine of the essence and the functioning conditions of this symbolising mechanism. I propose in this part of my book to start with what may be regarded as established, and then to take my readers by way of the probable, to the merely theoretical and hypothetical. I want to emphasise that I shall denote the whole pictorial and dramatising method of dream representation by the word "symbolic". (In general life, this term is used to denote a representation whose meaning is accessible to conscious thinking without much effort.) Further, Freud stresses in his writings that a certain group of "constant" symbols must be separated from the general pictorial mode of dream representation. We do not adhere to this distinction (from reasons understandable later). We are concerned mainly with the *fact of substitute-formation* and with the presumable cause and background, or the intrinsic meaning of such substitution and pictorial representation. Whether in any given case, we are dealing with a comparatively constant type of substitution, or whether this substitute is of a more individual, variable type, that is for our exposition merely a matter of detail. We shall come back to

this question when describing Freud's conception of dream interpretation.

(4) As the starting-point of our investigation we may conveniently choose a dream caused by an *organic stimulus*. *The synchronism and the close relation between the representation and that which is represented, is here comparatively obvious.* I think also that we may gain from this particular type of dream some enlightening aspects for the whole problem of the dream. The following dream-image is well qualified to serve as an illustration because of its simple structure :

> **12.** I have the urge to urinate. A man allows me to get on a bus which will take me to the nearest toilet permissible for me. He mounts the same bus and tells me where to alight. When I get there and enter, I find on trying to urinate that *the bowl is full.* I wake up and feel a strong urge to urinate.

Let us put ourselves in the place of the man, who, arriving after all his troubles in front of the full bowl, wants to urinate. On thus putting myself into such a situation, at once the feeling of " difficulty " has overcome me ; I felt that urination under such circumstances is extremely difficult, only possible if one ran the risk of making the bowl overflow. It is hard to avoid the suggestion that the full bowl is the pictorial representation of the *full and extended bladder*, an interpretation which would be in agreement with the symbolism of Scherner, for whom dreams are only representations of bodily processes. The motive implied in the whole situation—that there will be an overflow if he should urinate—may represent an exhortation not to take the dream as reality, and be so misguided by the hallucination as to wet the bed. Of course, if we thus interpret the bowl as a representation of the full bladder, it ceases to fit in properly with the rest of the dream, because now it represents not the " receiving part ", but its antithesis.

There is, however, another more satisfactory interpretation : that what is actually expressed in the dream is the feeling of strong urgency and the present difficulty of satisfying it without any risk. Let us visualise the events experienced in the dream. The dreamer feels a strong urge ; he has to go a long way before he can reach the toilet (where he can " alight ", i.e., urinate). But when getting there, it appears that his trip and expectation were futile because the bowl is full. The satisfaction of his need cannot take place, even by means of a dream-hallucination, since the real, unceasing tension within the bladder continually emphasises the non-fulfilment of the urge ; the " mindful " control of the sphincter muscle continues even during sleep. I think this more " completed " interpretation of the dream is at any rate acceptable ; the dream-situation, as analysed here, is in its totality quite suitable to represent the state of tension and distress as actually experienced.

(5) The first interpretation we gave of the dream-motif should, however, not be rejected. In accordance with everything we know of dreams, it is very unlikely that organic stimuli or other external events are simply " photographed " in the dream ; even the full content of a more or less complicated dream stimulated by an organic process, is *never* furnished exclusively by the physiological stimulus concerned. Experimental stimuli applied to the sleeper, appear more or less recognisable in the resulting dream-image, but they hardly account for all the remaining elements of the dream. The respective experiments of Maury are sufficiently known and are reported in Freud's *Interpretation of Dreams*. The following instance is one of this series. A drop of water is poured on the forehead of the sleeper ; his dream runs :

> **13.** He is in Italy, sweating heavily, and drinks white Orvieto wine.

An example which I had an opportunity to analyse and whose psychological background, therefore, was accessible to me, is the following : A friend of mine (occasionally my patient) was lying back on the sofa on a hot afternoon, reading. On the other end of the sofa was his wife, in a half-reclining position. He went to sleep, but could not stretch himself comfortably and freely, because his wife took up part of the sofa. He dreamt :

> **14.** I am sitting on the sofa with my wife and my uncle. There seems to be little room on the sofa, and I ask my wife to move over ; or was it my uncle who asked her to do this ?

We need spend no time on the obvious dream representation of the inconvenient position, and of the wish that the wife would not take up so much space. The closer consideration of the uncle in the dream-scene helps greatly in the correct understanding of the case. Originally, this uncle had been very much opposed to the marriage of my friend, his reason

being that she had not enough money ; in spite of his otherwise idealistic outlook, this uncle had a pathological regard
for financial means, a bank-balance outlook. In the dream,
there is an obvious allusion to this question of marriage ;
to the question of how far the uncle had been right ; . . .
how much the wife actually has furthered or limited the
career of the husband. This interpretation could be substanti-
ated when the dreamer added that in the dream the wife had
appeared uglier than she was in reality (underestimation),
and that actually at that period she was making a nuisance
of herself by her unjustified reproaches. This example may
convince even the most sceptical critic of dream analysis
about the true relation of the organic stimulus to the other
psychic sources.[1]

We are justified then in looking upon the bowl as the
representation of the full bladder, and yet in interpreting the
dream in its totality, as *a representation of the difficult subjective
situation of the dreamer*.[2] It is true, of course, that in this case
the full bladder and the difficulties of the dreamer, which
he cannot surmount during sleep, are closely and intrinsically
related to each other (cause and consequence). Essentially,
however, the dream depicts the actual psychic condition,
expressing the awareness of the relevant circumstances and
also the conscious fear of wetting the bed. (The rest of the
latent content is not considered here, although it has been
discovered.) *It is the attitude taken by the ego towards the organic
stimulus, the influence of the stimulus in question on the ego and the
social regard of the ego, which are represented in the dream-image.*

(6) Every organic stimulus which, in virtue of its intensity,
projects from the constant and normal unity of the " self-
feeling ", may be regarded as a miniature illness. Yet, illness
means : to *feel* ill. Every organic disturbance represents for
the psyche a disturbance of the ego-feeling. It is difficult to
know exactly in what this disturbance consists ; it is definitely
a complex psychoaffective event, the significance of which is
not exhausted by the mere perception of the anatomical-
physiological facts. We cannot tell precisely (can hardly
imagine in its full implications) what an organic event at
any given moment means for the personality ; how that
particular self-perception may fit in, at that time, with the
remainder of the psychoaffective structure. Stimulation,

---

[1] Cf. Ch. XII (13), (14).   [2] Cf. Ch. XII, dreams 91, 92, 93.

caused by pressure within the bladder, is always *the same to conscious perception* ; so is genital stimulation, or pain (apart from its certain qualitative and quantitative differences). But the endopsychic reaction, the effect of the perception of the stimulus on the psyche, is always different, because, in consequence of the multitude of other factors, the reacting psyche is not the same from moment to moment. (Similarly, the urge to urinate is different in its social import, when it can be appeased in safety, from what it is when it has to be repressed for one or two hours because of some environmental circumstances.) The state of the psyche, then, becomes changed in different ways and to varying degrees, by any organic stimulus, such as urinary, sexual or pain stimuli, perceived at any given particular moment by the psyche. In any case, the dream represents the state of our ego, which implies always a complex condition. We are now in the position to answer the question—at least in a provisional manner —why does an organic stimulus find a pictorial and scenic representation in the dream ? Because there is always *a composite psychic state* which would not be expressed properly if the dream said simply : " I am suffering pain ", or " I am hungry ", or " I badly want to urinate ". Even the actually scenic representation, of course, gives only a cross-section, a partial picture of the complete endopsychic state of affairs.

(7) Thus far we could only show the causes for the transformation of the organic stimulus into a wider kind of scene. Yet we have not explained by this why the scenic representation, this description of the endopsychic state of affairs, has to be carried out in symbolic, substitute-pictures, which are, at first, unrecognisable.

Now we know that in the dream we cited as an illustration, the difficulty of the objective and subjective situation, and the suffering of the experiencing person, are characterised by both the urgency (and the unsuccessfulness) of the long trip, and by the *full bowl*. But why this indirect, this allegorical representation ? Why could the situation not be represented by a scene, by a dream-experience, which might be described something like this :

> **15.** I feel the necessity to urinate, I try to find a toilet, but I notice that I am really lying in bed and cannot, therefore, get up and move about. I do not want, however, to wet the bed. My bladder is full, and hurts . . .

˙ It is obvious from all the dreams, caused by organic stimuli, that the dream-ego is ignorant of the actual position of the dreamer, of being asleep, and in bed ; after all, the dreamer lives and moves in variously coloured surroundings and goes through different experiences, like a person in waking state. (The rare exceptions to this rule are brought about by superficial, half-awake sleep.) The *scs.*, and consequently, the dreaming-ego, is not asleep, is not lying in bed, but is living through its kaleidoscopic adventures. *For this reason alone it is not possible for the dream to express the true condition of the personality.* This impossibility, and the fact implied in it, proves a fundamental thesis, which constitutes one of Freud's discoveries, viz., that dreaming, as such, is independent of the organic stimulus ; that the dreamer is already in his world of dreams at the moment when the organ-stimulus occurs as an added complication. It is, of course, true that we cannot tell for certain, what conceptual form the dream would have taken *in the absence* of the organic stimulus. But all other dreams which treat obviously and chiefly of the psychic problems of our waking life, of our recent difficulties, fears and hopes, prove sufficiently that the dream-content, as such, is *not* caused by the disturbing or normal organic stimulus. This was, however, actually maintained by Scherner, according to whom all dream-images are only " transformation-products " of organ-processes. We can point here to Silberer's well-known experiments, in which he demonstrated and proved that thoughts preceding sleep, reappear immediately in the dream-images (these experiments are dealt with in greater detail below) ; also to his findings that although in hypnagogic dreams (i.e., dream-like hallucinatory images experienced in the transition from waking state to sleep) the state of the body or its members constitutes one part of the material, the rest of the dream-content has definitely a different, a psycho-genic derivation. All this is sufficiently known and generally admitted, and there is no need to stress it. If then the dream-ego, at any rate and from quite different causation, has found itself in an " active, experiencing " state, the organic stimulus, suddenly emerging during sleep, naturally has to undergo a suitable transformation, so that it can be fitted into the continuity of the dream-experience. One cannot very well dream that one is walking about merrily, and to perceive in the same dream suddenly, upon the emergence of the urination-urge, that one is in bed, asleep, and must not wet the bed-clothes. Such an "illogical" change of scene may happen at times, but then it usually signifies some different psychic content, not simply a real bodily stimulus. The dreamer would have to wake up and to stop moving about in his dream-world in order to perceive the real nature of his urge to urinate. Otherwise, as pointed above, there must be an adapting transformation in the feature of the perceived stimulus. *This then is the second step in our approach, to explain the possible causes for the transformation of the organic stimulus into an imaginary picture.* I am, of course, conscious that we have been dealing here with an urge, which cannot be easily assuaged during sleep. (Vide Ch. VI.)   Yet it is not quite so easy to understand in the same way, why organic stimuli of a different kind—tactile, enteral, or auditory, etc.—are to be markedly transformed. One *could* walk and experience different events in the dream and at the same time could suddenly feel (within the same dream story) pains, or a tactile stimulus, and so on.

(8) In turning to the simultaneously occurring psychogenic dream event, which is independent of the additional organic stimulation, we have only shifted the problem to some extent. For, we find, as is well known, that the purely mental elements in the dream in most cases *also* show a changed, pictorial representation (Silberer's "functional phenomenon"). The interesting observations made by Silberer, and the considerable amount of confirmatory material available from analyses, proves this beyond question. (I think it is not superfluous to demonstrate inductively the correctness of this view, though it has been regarded as obvious. Freud's exposition on symbolism and "meaning" of the dream-elements is also essentially only dialectical, argumentative; he does not follow nor unfold the phenomenon in its development.) When one is on the verge of falling asleep and forces himself to gather his mind and to recollect the hypnagogic pictures experienced, it is often possible to recognise quite clearly trains of thought which originated in the period before sleep. "I am thinking before sleep about a problem," reports Silberer, "and cannot call to mind one particular detail." This is the resulting hypnagogic dream picture :

> 16. I ask for information in some office ; a bad-tempered secretary, who seems to have mislaid the relevant file, refuses to give it to me.

The relation is obvious between the mislaid file and the information refused in the dream, and the thought which Silberer could not call to his mind before the dream.

In another instance, the author tells about a visit to the theatre, where Faust was being played. " After going to bed, my thoughts are still occupied with the play. In spite of the overwhelming feeling of sleepiness, I try to concentrate on the difficult problem of the ' Mütter ' (mothers) which has caused so much heartbreak to interpreters of Goethe's work. Sleep finally overcomes me, the train of thought is suddenly broken, and in its place comes the following hallucination :

17. I am standing on a *solitary* promontory projecting far into the *dark* sea. The waters of the sea seem to blend with the dark sky, which is mysteriously heavy.

When I awake the picture vanishes. I recollect my previous train of thought and recognise that the hypnagogic dream was a symbol for the previous thoughts. The interpretation : My *solitary standpoint* indicates the remoteness of the problem, and the dark colouring of the picture, its darkness, its obscureness. The blending of sea and sky, the disappearance of the border between ' above and beneath ' was the symbol for the fact that in the problem treated of in the play, all time and space coalesce, so that Mephistopheles can say to Faust in the play : ' Sink down, then ! Or I might equally well say—Rise ! ' "

Let me cite a hypnagogic dream-imagery of my own. During a difficult period of my life, owing to the political circumstances in Czechoslovakia, I went to bed at night, saying to myself : " I can't bear it any longer." In the hypnagogic hallucination :

18. I see first of all an old Slovak man who is toiling laboriously cutting wood ; his undulating *locks* hide a face covered with sweat. Then I see a heroic figure from a film I once saw ; he is the hero of the Slovak people ; he fought gloriously against the suppressors of his brethren, and he was shown in the film dying in a last heroic fight. I see him rise proudly from his fetters and shake his *locks*. Lastly, I see some prone figure (dead ?). Perhaps it is my father (with a *beard* ?). This latter picture is not in accord with past reality. The meaning content seems to be quite simple : " this life with its struggle leads to final exhaustion, to an early death ". I may add that in my youth I used to say with regard to some difficult task that " it was as difficult as cutting wood ". . . .

A patient I once analysed was thinking before falling asleep of the varying course of the analytical hours. He experiences in the subsequent hypnagogic vision :

19. That a balloon or Zeppelin is rising ; a fighter zooms down.

My interpretation was : Two tendencies are alternating in his mind ; that towards superficiality and evasion (resistance, flight reflex), and the other one, towards deep analysis and the determination to " fight it out ".

Here, too, the mutual relation is fairly clear. Besides, we notice as in the case of the organ-sensation dreams, the change, the pictorial transformation and at the same time " a widening" of the thought-content. In this dream picture we find expressed *not only* the fact that the analytical sessions have varying success (ups and downs), but also the decision, based on recognition of the necessity, to dare *to delve down into the depths,* in order to regain health and to be able again to dwell on the ground of " earthy reality ".

I may say the same with regard to my own hypnagogic dream. The pictures while symbolising my state at that time, imply also that I was a hero, a fighter, and a victim of the circumstances. Indeed, that very day I had thought about the impossibility of publishing my best work because of the adverse political conditions, and how I should not be able to go on with my scientific experiments. The continuation of my dream related it to the figure of my father, who in the course of his duties as a clergyman, at one period also had *to fight* hard for his principles. I also remembered in this connection that my father, who was ignorant of the Slovak language (at that time Slovakia was part of Hungary), could make himself understood only *with difficulty* to the Slovak workers and woodcutters, who were working in our house. It is clear that the associations to my dream are not simply associations by similarity or true relationship, but *completions* of the content of my vision, necessary adjuncts to the description of the dream.   (I have omitted several other associations and aspects of analytical importance.)

(9) We ask now again : Whence this tendency towards dramatisation and personification of our thoughts and feelings ? The bad-tempered secretary obviously depicts the annoying forgetfulness, as well as the realisation that the dreamer himself

was not responsible for the failure to remember that one detail.

The fighter 'plane represents the desirable positive attitude towards the analytical treatment. In my own case it is the struggle, the at present thwarted ambition, which is personified by the various figures (one might speak, though inaccurately, of identification). In Silberer's second example, it is the difficulty and vastness of the problem, and the condition of the contemplating mind, which is symbolised through a natural scene.

It is obvious, both from the organic dreams described earlier, as well as from the above mentioned " autosymbolic dreams " (Silberer) that the sleeping and dreaming ego conceives of the psychical and physical stimuli in a fashion different from that of the waking-ego. As long as psychology has regarded and considered *only* the various disturbing physical stimuli during sleep, it was possible to speak of misinterpretation of their true nature by the sleeping-ego, and of a kind of error, i.e., illusion. Yet it is very difficult to regard the transformation of thought-contents, and even of thinking processes, as the result of illusions, because—I want to stress this particularly —the processes and contents of thinking have always their subconscious, unconscious roots, and it is clearly impossible in this connection to speak of " misinterpretation " in the sense of illusion. It is true, we said that it is rather " conditions, states " of the psyche and the body which are transformed in the dream. But in the examples given above, it is well-nigh impossible to separate the thought-content from the respective condition. Purely descriptively it might be spoken of as a misinterpretation of the state of affairs in general. *But psychologically we must assume that the respective self-perception has actually a different meaning and content for our sleep and dream-consciousness.* The question now is this : are the feelings only personified for the purpose of dream representation, or are they really experienced in the same or similar manner in which they appear represented ? I admit that it is difficult to accept this latter alternative, with everything that it implies, and to say : " Yes, the dream-ego experiences the stimulus or the thought that moves us, really as if it were a person, a thing, a locality, an objective scene. But to accept the other alternative would mean to attribute an unbelievable primitiveness to the human psychic apparatus, and to assume that there are mere playful and nonsensical pictorial dream-representations, accompanying the completely unchanged self-perceptions.

(10) I should like to advance the following hypothesis, at first briefly formulated, which will later on be supported by arguments and by references to empirical observations :

Stimuli and processes of our *inner world* are perceived *differently* by the dream-ego and by the waking-ego. A different state of the psyche implies a different mode of perception. When in the dream-image organic, emotional and thought-events are represented in the form of images, and are objectified as things and persons, that must be interpreted as suggesting that these perception-elements *have a different form and a different content for our dream-consciousness, as compared with the waking consciousness.* Although I do not want to maintain, much less to prove, that in dream 12 the full bladder really appeared to the *scs.* and to the dream-ego as a full bowl, or in dream 16 the forgotten thought as a bad-tempered secretary, *yet the appearance of the substitute-idea in the dream implies that the respective self-perception by the* scs. *and dream-consciousness was essentially different from the perception and idea of the waking consciousness.* If a particular mental element were identical in content for the *scs.* and the dream-ego on the one hand, and for the waking consciousness on the other, probably its dream-representation would also be unchanged. What appears unchanged to the *scs.* and to the dream-ego, reaches the dream-image in the form customary to waking thought. This accounts for the peculiar mixture in our dreams of elements characteristic of the waking system of conceptual thinking, and of those characteristic of the substitute-forming symbolic system ; a fact to which we have already drawn attention, and which statement must have appeared at first sight no more than a confusing and arbitrary assumption.[1]   Toothache, the urge to relieve nature, hunger, thirst and libidinous desire, once they reach a certain insistence, appear in the dream more obviously recognisable, because these stimuli are, in virtue of their intensity, more likely to retain their waking quality, even during the formation of the dream ; it seems almost as if these minor stimuli interrupt momentarily the deep, proper sleep, only to give way again to these deeper levels, and to the proper dream-phenomena, pertaining thereto. The total

[1] Cf. p. 25.

content of the dream, however, is then synthesized by the secondary " conceptualising " function, and formed into *one* homogeneous dream containing both elements.

(11) It is easy to see these mechanisms at work, in a group of dreams described by Rank in his paper on " Levels of Symbol-Formation in Dreams " ; (quoted by Freud, *Interpretation of Dreams*, Ch. VI). One can observe in some cases, that a certain physical stimulus appears in the dream at first more or less intensely disguised, then, as the irritation becomes stronger and the sleep less profound, the dream-representation of the stimulus is more obvious and recognisable. It was actually Scherner who recognised and rightly interpreted this phenomenon. A pollution-dream of a patient I once analysed, may render the discussion more concrete :

> **20.** I am looking for a room, but *I don't want the caretaker to see me*. I open a door very *cautiously* ; I then see a *woman* whose look I like, but *I am shy to betray this to her*. Suddenly I have the feeling that *I have slept with her* . . . I wake up and am aware that *ejaculation* is taking place.

In the first part of the dream there is only a room (well-known Freudian symbol for a woman), and the timidity associated with the presence of the caretaker. Overtly, in the second part, there is already a woman, and the feeling of bashfulness, which prevents the dreamer from showing interest in her. The final part is formed subjectively by the clear awareness of the past actual erotic event, and objectively by the pollution.

Another very interesting organic dream also belongs to this type. A man of 45, who had sought my advice because of peculiar constricting pains in his chest, told me of his dream experienced during an attack of his pains :

> **21.** I am driving through a narrow, winding street in a strange car. A tyre bursts, and I have to repair it. Another car wants to pass, and I have to jump on the foot-board of my car, thus getting caught between the two vehicles. I wake up suddenly with a cry ; my chest and my head hurt badly.

The relation between the *narrowness* of the street in the dream, and the *constricting pain in the chest* is obvious. I know nothing about the dreamer ; I saw him only twice and could not make up my mind whether he was suffering from an organic trouble (angina pectoris or tabes), or whether his pains had a functional origin (vascular spasms). If we assume that the two vehicles represent conflicting psychic tendencies, causing a pathological reaction of the vascular system, we can understand the dream in its entirety. The driving in a strange car and the recognition of the necessity to make room for the other car, could be easily interpreted on this basis. (The dreamer might be a bearer of a complex, " strange " to his conscious ego, attempting to avoid the " conflict " collision and to repair the existing damage ; the interpretation might run on these or similar lines.)   But I want to consider the dream in these cases only as an organ-sensation dream.   I assume that the painful attack was dreamed as it developed, as it grew more painful. First, we have the narrow, winding street which was explained above as originating from the constriction ; then the break-down of the car which might still possibly be repaired, this representing the hope that the attack might decrease in intensity and cease altogether ; the attempt to let the other car pass, is again another symbolic expression of the same hope ; finally, at the end of the dream, comes the accident in all its seriousness, i.e., the manifest representation by the dream of the fully developed constricting pain in the chest.

What is the true nature of this sort of dream-picture ?   We know that the duration of dreams in general, and of organic dreams in particular, is short ; I do not believe that in these two cases a slow and long development of the irritation has been represented. It is more likely that the gradual and closer approximation of the dream-representation to the objective facts and their realistic perception was caused by a lessening of the depth of sleep in consequence of the irritation by the stimulus.   Let us consider the first example.   As long as the timidity and bashfulness in the dream (a sentiment which, as revealed by the latent content, covered serious inhibitions) has not been overcome and disregarded, *the instinctual drive itself, in its objectivity, must have been modified ; it means not only weakened in intensity, but changed in its very quality.* (In the *subconscious* there is no qualifying without essential alteration.) This would be *one* way of interpreting this dream-phenomenon. Another interpretation would be, that during deep sleep the stimulus, the erotic tendency was at first not recognised in its true nature ; as waking thinking was gradually reached, this recognition became feasible.   In the second example it is hardly possible to speak of an " overcoming " of an " inhibition ".   At the most, one might assume a tendency, to maintain undisturbed sleep and to annul the disturbing influences (this would be similar to Freud's " convenience-dreams " which try to render the urgent getting up unnecessary, and to ensure undisturbed sleep). A second possibility, here too, would be that the growing pain-intensity was actually appreciated only gradually, yet without any attempt of active hallucinatory annulment of its perception. I think that both interpretations in the two cases enable us in assuming that : Whatever is not perceived by the dream-ego in keeping with the mode of waking thinking, becomes represented by the dream figuratively. Conversely, *whatever appears in the dream in a pictorial, figurative fashion, has been for the scs., at least at the time of dreaming, and accordingly for the dream-ego, an already modified psychic element.*

(12) This may be shown also by another group of dreams, namely those in which an event concerning the dreamer, is *displaced* on to another person. During the evening and also during sleep, I was suffering from a kind of rheumatic pain in the region of the *right* scapula. I dreamed :

> **22.** Mrs. R. rushes quickly into my consulting-room and asks to be examined. She then says : " You were on the point of leaving." I agree, as it is almost seven, and dinner will soon be served. I am annoyed that, in spite of this, she insists on an examination. I take my stethoscope and examine her. But suddenly it is an elderly, rather thin man whose reflexes I examine with a hammer. He appears to be, in the dream, the husband of Mrs. R. She is also present, and then the landlady comes in. I percuss around the *left* clavicle and ask if he feels any pain ; I suspect some chronic disease (of the lungs ?). He denies having pain there and points to his *right* shoulder, where earlier on I had heard some suspicious sounds. I wake up with bad pains in the same region. (I was supposed to get up at 7 a.m. to carry out an analysis ; cf. the 7 o'clock in the dream.)

The day before an unknown woman had called at my home, to ask me to recommend her to prospective boarders. I thought her loud and obtrusive. Mrs. R., on the other hand, although perhaps a trifle loud, is a woman I like quite well. She also keeps boarders. The mistress of the house, formerly also a practising physician, earns her living similarly by taking in boarders. I have the impression that she is not satisfied with the amount of money I pay her, although I know that it is not customary to pay more. These associations are cited only to explain, though rather superficially, my unsympathetic feeling towards Mrs. R. which is displayed in the dream.

Now let us turn to the pain, and to its displacement to another person. The figure of the man reminds me of an extremely emaciated but very ambitious and industrious patient I once had, and also of *my* lassitude at that time. In addition, he reminds me of the success of my efforts then. The identification is clear. What is the significance of the displacement? One is hardly justified in refusing the most straightforward explanation. *If the pain is attacking somebody else, then I am healthy. If I am using the stethoscope and hammer, then I am again a freely-practising doctor, not a refugee in England,* who at first, is allowed to practise psychotherapy, but not his equally loved and even much more remunerative neurology. I mention this latter aspect also to stress and to support the wish-fulfilling tendency of the displacement of the pain. A history is also attached to the area on the left side, which I tap suspiciously in the dream. I am very much afraid now of the slightest cold, because it might bring back the neuralgic pain in the same region which caused me so much trouble last winter ; not so much through its intensity as through the difficulties it put in the way of my newly formed practice and by limiting my walks, exercises, etc. By *denying* the existence of pain on this spot, I am relieved of my anxiety. I have always maintained that transformation and displacements in dreams, represent *attempts at cure* (when, for instance, one's own pathological complex is displaced on to some other person, etc.). Such an attempt would be quite meaningless, if the element concerned were not itself, in its essence, really transformed for the *scs*. Dreaming is a biological function. (Cf. Ch. X).

Just as wishfulfilment, taking place in the dream, is a true satisfying *experience*, not simply a self-deceptive *illusion* (cf. Ch. VI on Food-Dreams), so displacement, and all similar mechanisms of disguise within the dream-event, are signs of a partial or attempted transformation, which make easier the bearing of the facts, i.e., either of an organic illness or of a complex, endangering psychic harmony.[1]

(13) This group of dreams—and other examples will follow —illustrates clearly : (1) that the psychic element (in this

[1] Cf. Ch. III (34).

case the pain-sensation, and the knowledge of it), is being transformed in the direction of that which is easier and more endurable, in the sense of diminution of its painful quality ; (2) that, therefore, there is a biological tendency quite definitely implied in the dream-transformations ; (3) that though the transformed dream-element is reducible to a conscious element, to a real perception (in our case of an organic event), yet psychologically the " symbol " or " picture " coincides with a new, transformed element in the *scs.*, and does not correspond congruently with the original or conscious perception. Schematically, we might put it in the following way : First comes the real pain (in waking state we would have to add the conscious perception of that pain) ; secondly, there is a weakening of the pain, brought about by the state of sleep ; thirdly, there is the dream-representation of this feeling, as it is being perceived in its weakened form. *Displacement is the result.*

The same process may be illustrated by the following example. The dreamer is suffering from precordial pains which were diagnosed as functional angina, due to exhaustion of the heart-muscle in consequence of continuous mental and physical exertion.

> **23.** My brother, from a high ladder, falls *headlong* ; he is stunned, but recovers soon, and finds that nothing serious has happened to him. The dreamer wakes up with a moderate feeling of anxiety.

Here the feeling of anxiety, caused by the condition of the heart, appears to have been subjected to the process of *objectification*. The dreamer's own " organic " anxiety receives a quasi-justification in the dream by his frightened reaction to the accident of his brother. This accident of the brother in the dream carries, however, obviously the meaning of " serious danger ", of " bodily injury ". Thus the dream, in its detailed composition, may be regarded as a displacement-dream. (There is also a second kind of displacement, i.e., from the heart to the *head*, which change possibly indicates the *nervous* nature of the distress. Can this be considered as a point of diagnostic value, or merely as the patient's sub-conscious attempt at self-pacification ?) We know other types of dreams in which the objectification of one's own fear occurs *without* displacement. For instance, a woman suffering badly from attacks of genuine angina pectoris, dreamt one night, when she was not feeling very well :

24. There was some talk of a *poisoned goose*, and the question was discussed whether one might eat it or not. I wake up with anxiety.

It is possible that the poisoned goose signifies the dreaming person herself, in her being ill, thus constituting some kind of *displacement* of her own suffering to another object ; of course, in the question of whether one might eat the meat, there is contained still a reference to her own person.[1] The following dream, however, shows beyond doubt the mechanism of pure objectification, of personification of the dreamer's own distress due to an attack of cardiac asthma : the danger to life is referred overtly to the dreamer's *own ego*, transformed only in its character and weakened through the particular explanation advanced for it, in the dream :

25. Two shadowy figures, burglars, attack the dreamer ; he tries to escape to a neighbouring room. He wakes up with feelings of fear and can hardly breathe.

Here the threatening anoxæmia is personified in the same manner as in the dream No. 16 where the dreamer's forgetfulness was personified by the secretary, who refused to give any information. In that example, too, we have seen how the disagreeable forgetfulness of the dreamer has been projected on to a figure, who is independent of the dreamer's will, i.e., the painful fact weakened and became transformed in the perception of the scs. ; (one is, after all, indeed not responsible for one's forgetfulness ; the dream displacement in such a case is certainly justified). In displacement-dreams this tendency of weakening, carried out by separation of the fact in question from the ego is, of course, quite clear. *Yet this tendency in the dream signifies most decidedly a transformation of the element of the perception in the* scs.

(14) This thesis finds support also in the displacement-dreams which have mainly a *psycho-affective* origin. Everyone who studies dreams, meets frequently with instances, in which the dreamer's own actions, wishes and strivings, as far as they are in opposition to his moral ego, are displaced on to others. An elderly spinster, who had avoided all erotic temptations though only with great effort, dreamt :

---

[1] Psychologically it is, of course, possible to assume that the pre-morbid, healthy personality regards the pain, or the anomaly, as foreign to its structure, and refuses at first to acknowledge it as its own.

26. My friend has turned frivolous ; she goes out with men at night.

We may look upon the " friend " as the symbol of the dreamer's libido ; or as the symbol of her genitals ; or we may regard the whole dream simply as a displacement of that kind which sometimes happens in real life, namely, when one uncritically displaces one's own feelings and tendencies on to others. Whichever formula of interpretation we choose, we can hardly deny the qualifying transformation of the original drive. Young girls who, after puberty, start to feel the strength of the sexual drive, often have dreams of a similar kind. Sometimes also they dream of men who pursue them in order to catch, to beat or to stab them. We consider this latter type of dreams and the accompanying feelings of fright and anxiety, as related to the mechanism of repression, consequent upon the moral struggle. *In all these cases it is clear that we must suppose a true, essential transformation of the repressed mental elements ; otherwise we could ascribe no useful purpose to the process of repression.* When drives and tendencies encounter resistance from the moral ego, the ensuing struggle signifies the attempt, to render these drives relatively harmless, inactive, by transforming their essential qualities. Sublimation is only *one* possible way and result of this deep process of metamorphosis. I find it hardly possible to think of any weakening-process in the *scs.* which does not imply an essential transformation. We may consider here a chemical analogy : salicylic acid is transformed by only slight structural changes into the different acetylosalicylic acid (aspirin) which latter is much more suited for general consumption. When, then, in such cases, as previously mentioned, the instinctual drive appears in the dream as the pursuer, it is comprehended by the psyche, correctly, as something foreign and strange in character to the ego-ideal. The displacement occurring in these dreams is due then, in fact, to the essential transformation in the *ucs.* of the psychic element or complex in question. We refer here to a deeper unconscious level of the ego, because we are dealing with a substantial transformation of instinctive drives, and must assume that such processes occur at deeper levels than the " subconscious " ones which are brought into play in connection with the repression of higher conceptual elements.

(15) The closer one has approached the problem of dreams

and the more experience one has gained, one might even say the more one has learned to " live " in the world of dreams —the more one comes to appreciate that there is *no* heterogeneity of dreams ; that the fundamental mechanisms at work are *not* so multiform, as the different events, represented in the dreams, might lead one to suppose. I believe, we are fully justified in applying certain conclusions, drawn from *one* group of dreams, to another ; we are justified in transferring insight gained from one group to others ; as long as in doing so we do not limit the field of our investigations and interpretations. When it is obvious in one group of dreams, that behind the pictorial, symbolic representation there is an element which has been *transformed* in the *scs.*, we are perhaps safe in concluding reversely from the fact that some organic or psychic event *is* represented in a symbolical fashion in the dream, that this particular mental element pre-existed in the *scs.* in a transformed, essentially changed state. (Cf. p. 40.)

In the case of physiological, organic stimuli which impinge upon the sleeper, a *different* perception is obvious, because of the very fact of the sleeping state. Apart from this, the stimulation itself is extending into a complicated psychic element, as for instance, in the quoted dream about an urge to urinate, where the whole condition of the dreamer is represented (" I want to, but I can't, and it is very painful "). In the case of pain or of a repressed tendency, the content is being transformed for obvious reasons. In the dreams with " levels of symbol formation " the different types of perception on the different levels of the sleeping state are quite clear. We may add that it is only reasonable to assume that a subconscious element, compared with its conscious counterpart, is being in some way transformed, extended, and fitted into the whole structure of the *scs.* The predominance of pictorial and symbolic representations in the dreams points in all probability to the different nature of subconscious elements. I am aware of the fact, of course, that this conclusion from the material assembled above, is not logically unassailable. It might, e.g., be maintained that the dream-work gravitates towards a figurative mode of representation for reasons not precisely accountable, and treats, therefore, all the material offered by the *scs.* in the same pictorial and symbolical way, whether or not it has undergone an essential transformation there, as compared to its original conscious counterpart. Yet, this apparently cautious, would-be objective manner of looking at the facts, bars the way to further progress and to greater insight. *I believe that we can and should derive conclusions from conditions such as are obviously present in some groups of dreams, and make these conclusions obtain for the working of the dream in general.*

The process of dreaming is a function of the psyche, of the nervous system, and every such function is carried out by mechanisms and in ways which are uniform in their very nature (cf. Ch. X on " The Biological Status of Dreaming ".) Otherwise we would have to postulate the existence of senseless events, void of understandable causation and purpose, instead of gaining a unifying, generally valid point of view. A true sense of science demurs at such fruitless and limiting objectivity ; at a passive acceptance of a view which would render quite meaningless and irregular such a constant psychic phenomenon as the dramatisation and the symbolic transformation of contents by the dream work ; a view which would regard as incapable of further explanation what is, one can say, the main characteristic feature of such a constant life phenomenon as dreaming. The mere reference to " old, archaic mechanisms " as the only source of symbolism in dreams, is surely too inadequate, and quite insufficient to explain the significance of a process of such a high order.

I lay so much stress on the point in question for certain reasons of principle. I have in mind those psychologists who for sentimental reasons cannot agree with the too simple " mechanistic " conception of the *scs. All theories* regarding the nature of the *scs.* are, of course, *pure speculations* ; while the existence of the Freudian libidinous drives is a more palpable reality. In spite of this it must be said that the original classical psychoanalytic conception of the unconscious, in its relation to the dream, is too " mechanistic " and schematic.[1] That much will be admitted more or less freely, by every investigator of the younger analytic generation. And the limited fashion of interpretation of the dream-content which is based on this conception, will satisfy fewer and fewer analysts, especially those who are in need of a shortened time-saving method of psychotherapy. This is not meant as polemics ; I think that in my description and discussion

[1] Cf. Ch. VI.

E

of Freud's dream-theory I show clearly my desire to be, as far as possible, unbiased. Yet I believe at the same time that in matters concerning the psyche, even sentimental motives and counter-arguments may be of some positive value. Moreover, practical psychotherapy shows a real need for a more flexible technique of interpretation. In the passive, but long, classical psychoanalysis much is being solved, relieved and cured spontaneously, though not spoken of, and not dealt with directly (this being the effect of time and transference factor). In the shortened, so-called active forms of psychotherapy, such neglect of important psychic contents and aspects is not permissible. Quite naturally, I could not contribute anything new and valuable by my present arguments and general explanations to the " philosophy " of the unconscious. I wanted only to indicate that the unconscious should be looked upon as being more than the place of repression ; and should not be considered merely as the obscure region of instinctive drives. And thus the dream, and its symbolic mode of representation, contains more by far than the limited interpretations of classical psychoanalysis have allowed us to surmise. Above all, we have gathered evidence of the richness of the " *functional* " *elements* in the dream.[1] The remark made above about the spontaneous curative effect of a long-lasting classical analysis answers the possible question how such a passive method may still result in the successful treatment of certain symptoms without resorting to those different modern psychotherapeutic viewpoints suggested by pioneers of. psychological research.

(16) Freud's theory of dreams, which will be described and discussed later, submits as *one* possible mode of disguising the latent dream-content the symbolic transformation of elements. (Admittedly, he had in mind only certain special and fixed symbols which are connected with the representation of chiefly erotic contents and aggressive tendencies.) " Symbolism must be recognised as a second, independent mechanism of dream-representation, next in importance to the dream-censor. It might be surmised, however, that it is convenient for the dream-censor to make use of symbolism, since both mechanisms lead to the same end, i.e., the strangeness and incomprehensibility of the dream." (Freud : *Introductory Lectures.*) It is obvious, as seen in this quotation, that Freud does not

---

[1] Discussed later, Ch. III, pp. 78–84, and also in Ch. XII.

fundamentally reduce this mode of representation only to the tendency of the dream to disguise its genuine content. Elsewhere he writes : " One has the impression that we are dealing here with an old and extinct mode of work."

Freud reduces certain kinds of pictorial transformation in dreams (which he, however, separates from symbolism proper) to the tendency towards easier representation. " A colourless and abstract expression of the dream-thought is exchanged for one that is pictoria land concrete. The advantage, and along with it the purpose, of this substitution is obvious. Whatever is pictorial is more capable of representation in dreams, and can be fitted in to a situation in which an abstract expression would confront the dream-representation with difficulties, not unlike those which would arise, if a political editorial had to be represented in an illustrated journal." A lady dreams :

> 27. She is at the opera : in the middle of the stalls there is a *high tower*, on the top of which there is a platform surrounded by an iron railing. There stands the conductor continually running round behind the railing, perspiring terribly ; and from this position he is conducting the orchestra.

Freud interprets : " I knew that she had felt intense sympathy for a musician whose career had been prematurely brought to an end by insanity. *The man towered above all* the other members of the orchestra. This tower must be described as a composite formation by means of apposition ; by its structure it represents the *greatness* of the man, but the railing on the top behind which he runs around like a prisoner or an animal in a cage (an allusion to the name of the unfortunate man—Wulf), *represents his later fate*. ' Lunatic tower ' [1] is perhaps the expression in which the two thoughts might have met." (Extract from : *The Interpretation of Dreams*.)

Freud also admits that dreams sometimes contain *abstract thoughts* of the usual waking type ; i.e., that the dreamer in his dream simply knows or feels that someone is particularly great ; or that this knowledge finds expression in a directly formed thought and sentence. " Dreams then think preponderantly, but not exclusively, in visual images. They also make use of auditory images and to a lesser extent of the other sensory impressions. Moreover, in dreams, as in the waking state, many things are simply thought or imagined

[1] An old-fashioned expression for asylum.

(probably with the help of remnants of verbal conceptions). Characteristic of dreams, however, are *only* those elements of its content, which behave like images ; that is to say, which more closely resemble perceptions than mnemonic representations. We may say that the dream hallucinates, that it replaces thought by hallucinations. In this respect visual or acoustic impressions behave in the same way. It has been observed that the recollection of a succession of notes, heard as one is falling asleep, becomes transformed, after we have fallen asleep, into a lively hallucination of the same melody, to give place, each time we wake, to their fainter and qualitatively different representation of the memory, and resuming again each time we dose off again, its full hallucinatory character. From these images the dream creates a more complete situation which we are actually experiencing in dreaming."

(17) Little can be added to this classical description. I would like only to point out that dream-events may, however, be compared with those of waking life only in so far as we want to say that we *experience* in the dream, and not merely think, imagine and remember. But with equal certainty we must emphasise the subjectively perceptible difference in the quality of the two types of experiencing. Subjectively, the quality of the dream-experience is *not entirely* similar to that of waking life. The events appear to be more overwhelming, the scenes seem to concern one more closely, and deeply. Perhaps, because in the dream, *spectator and actor are one with the action.* In the real world, we feel more separated from our environment and the events taking place therein ; the " I " and " you " are more clearly defined and distinct to our subjective perception than is the case in the dreams. It might be added that the *spatial* character of events in dreams shows, with rare exceptions, a relatively narrow demarcation.[1] *Everything seems to point to the fact that essentially we are dealing with events occurring within the single, individual psyche, which are being represented by the multiform, colourful action of the dream ; that there is a unity behind the phenomenological complexity of dream-components* (such as are space, images, persons, actions, etc., of the dream-scene). We will return to this topic in Ch. V. Contrasting with this suggested actual unity of the total dream-event is the splitting up of the ego by the

[1] Cf. Ch. XII, dream 81.

dream-representation, the personification of its various components, of its drives, tendencies and sentiments.

(18) The reason usually given for this unreal, hallucinatory perception of inner events, for the dramatisation and personification of thoughts, feelings and physiological processes, is the *dissociation of psychic unity* during sleep. Thus Havelock Ellis says : " . . . the usually coherent elements of our mental life are split up and some of them—often it is curious to note, precisely those which are at that very moment the most prominent and poignant—are reconstituted into what seems to us an outside world." It cannot be denied, in spite of all our modern discoveries regarding the meaningfulness of dreams, that as compared with waking conscious thinking and judgment, we find mental functions during sleep definitely inferior, or at least inferior from a certain point of view. But, on the other hand, we must not rest content with the idea that any constant function of the wonderfully composed human organisation could be so useless, so " backward ", as the lack of our knowledge and especially that of the professional investigators of any given culture period might sometimes suggest. To apply this to the problem of dream interpretation : when one compares the degree of progress since the first tentative approach of Freud's psychoanalytic method with the state of affairs obtaining *before* that time (not to speak about the further progress he made later), one cannot but come to the conclusion that any assumption which in a purely negative manner simply states the " accidental ", and the irregularity in the various manifestations of life, can claim only a provisional validity. If we accept even a small fraction of the results of modern research on dreams as proved ; if we take the theories of Freud as only applicable to one certain fraction of the multitude of dreams (as does for instance the experienced and learned Havelock Ellis) ; if we accept only to a very limited degree the interpretations of Stekel, which at first seem so fantastic and purely intuitive, but which, nevertheless, proved very useful in practice (as does Freud in his turn) [1] ; if finally we add the interesting points of view of Jung, Adler, and all the others who have made valuable and suggestive contributions ; then it seems really short-sighted to put too much stress on the imperfect mode

---

[1] In Ch. VI (" The Dream-work "), and in the preface to the third German edition.

of the working of the dream. For, *before* the era of psycho-analytic investigations nearly everything in the dream-work seemed consequent upon the irregular, dissociated mode of the working of the dream-ego, and therefore not to be taken seriously. *The apparent unreal mode of the dream, and the dissociation of the psychic unity during sleep are undeniable facts. Yet they constitute mechanisms of their own, special methods of work, and not merely simply negative characters.* I expect the reader will shake his head disbelievingly and regard this latter statement as fantastic assumption, not warranted by anything. But the same happened when the public was confronted with the first of Freud's attempts and explanations. (The present author does not try, of course, to compare his small, though perhaps not quite valueless, contributions with Freud's great and far-reaching discoveries ; he wants only to recall to the reader the for us almost inconceivable " refusal to understand " and the expressions of astonishment which are to be found in the literature of that time.) A good deal of recent work which is being quoted and referred to in this volume, and all that is suggested with regard to the biological function of dreaming, show that we are fully entitled to look for regularity and significance even where objective science so far has been forced to halt.[1] I shall not pretend to be able to explain everything ; even science of future generations will not be able to accomplish this task. The miracle of life permits of partial insight only, of presentiments, but never of the real and " conquering " appropriation by means of deepest and fullest comprehension. What I want to stress, and ask the reader to accept, is the fundamental meaningfulness of all the phenomena of life, including those of dreaming. This anticipatory assumption is at least as likely to ensure progress as the objective, cautious and unbiased observation and investigation of mere details, of individual events, regarded apart from the whole of which they are only a constituent. What is it that unconsciously spurs on every investigator, if not this presentiment of the regular nature of phenomena, the presence of certain laws, of meaning in the multiformity of the world of our experiences ? Is it not this more or less unconscious feeling of the complete *unity of the universe* ?

---

[1] There are several problems, important for the theory and practice of dream-interpretation, which could be investigated on the basis of sufficient material. The present time gives no opportunity for such a work.

Truly, it is not illogical, at least it is intelligible, that the man of our era, trained and matured by the modern philosophy of natural science, also assumes the presence of a creative spirit, of a Deity behind this unity of phenomena, as a brilliant thinker, S. R. Hirsch has pointed out.

(19) Let us accept the dream-ego, with all its modes of work as a given phenomenon ; let us try to accustom ourselves to the idea that what happens in this sphere of psychic life must happen in *this* manner, in order to fulfil the natural aim and intrinsic purpose of the function in question ; that the phenomena which we encounter in this sphere, are in their own way as meaningful, as proper to the end in view as are waking thought and waking feeling. After all, we might ask with the same justification : What is the purpose in life of thinking? This question is too abstract, too theoretical and philosophical to be dealt with here ; nor is the present author qualified to discuss it. But the relation between dreaming (not as it is sometimes inaccurately called dream-thinking ; the phenomena are actually too complex to be subsumed under such a restricted term) and the thinking process proper, is too close to make it permissible to eschew entirely the question of the *psychobiological function of thinking*. It can hardly be doubted that it is part of " life " ; that it fulfils a corresponding function in life. It is responsible for the orientation of the personality in all its relations to the external world, and to one's own psycho-physiological world. But apart from this quality of *external usefulness* there is quite definitely also a " *pleasure-quality* " in the act of thinking, a kind of satisfaction of a need. The feeling of relief and of satisfaction, when one succeeds in giving conceptual form to a feeling, to an emotional content, is too well known to require detailed description here. If I may use the psychoanalytic phrase, there is *narcissistic cathexis of the total mental personality*. Perhaps a comparison with the satisfaction of hunger and sexuality may be illustrative. These two fields of functions serve the purpose of preservation of the self and preservation of the race respectively. But the performance of both instinctive functions is associated with such intense pleasure that one is surely justified in looking upon this gain of pleasure as a separate factor in life. Admittedly, the striving for æsthetically more pleasing food ensures the relative goodness of the food ; while similarly the striving for sexual pleasure

ensures survival of the race, and also the search for the stronger
or more beautiful mate possibly furthers the selection of
favourable heredity-factors. But striving on both fields for
the pleasurable has become in men so thoroughly autonomous,
that there is little doubt of the independent rôle of the search
for the beautiful and agreeable, within the frame of these
two great instinctive drives. Similarly the double function
of thinking : first, it exists in order to *safeguard life*, secondly
it serves as a psychic source of *pleasure*. Dreaming might
be understood in the same manner ; it is a satisfaction of a
need, of a special requirement of the organism.[1] This assumption may sound artificial and even poetical ; yet it is definitely
no more fantastic than the alternative assumption that the
existence of the world of dreams is something biologically
useless, and that the kind of dreaming as it is known to us,
is only a consequence of the dissociated function of the brain.
The biological status and significance of the deepest, non-
conceptual dream-processes will be dealt with in a later
chapter. Here we are interested rather in the question of
why the concept-formation in dreams takes such a pictorial
form. Although it is impossible to give an unequivocal, clear
answer, one may surmise the reason if one is not too much
biased in a negativistic direction. As the act of thinking in
its " pleasure-quality ", as that thinking which does not
subserve the orientation towards external reality, but meta-
morphoses continuously the psychic content for its own sake
(l'art pour l'art), thus dreaming, too, appears essential in life.
*The world of dreams appears as dissociated only in comparison with
the world of conscious thought*, in relation to the world of logical
reality. But why assume and take for granted that the world
of dreams wants to be compared with, and related to, the
world of reality and realistic thinking ? *The contrary is much
more probable. The world of dreams is a world apart.* One who
bears in mind the manifold dreams whose beauty reminds
one of fairy-tales, one who thinks of dream-scenes in which
problems of the day, sometimes important questions, are
dealt with in continuation of waking thinking ; of the subconscious continuation, and at times amazingly extensive
development of wishes, plans and cares of the waking life—
will only with hesitation " reproach " the dream-ego with its
comparative deficiencies, and reduce the formation of dreams

[1] Cf. Ch. XI, p. 185.

only to the negative factor of the cessation of the conscious thinking process.

(20) I want here to cite, though only briefly, two different theoretical constructions, which independently of each other deal respectively with the processes of thinking and the dramatic images of the dream world. The essential agreement between the two views seem here worthy of stress. Schilder, in his *Psychoanalytic Presentation of Psychiatry*, remarks very aptly that the significance of an *idea* lies in its immediate relation to *action*. But no idea is reached during the thought-process without first passing through several intermediate steps. Every thinking act has to work its way from the periphery of the idea to its centre, i.e., to the position of its clear and final completeness. Along this path lie the *symbolical* and other related intermediate products. Should the process encounter an " opposing impulse " which tends in a different direction, then there ensues a " halt " at the stage of a substitute-image. The image produced in this manner is not as near to the sphere of action as is the idea proper. Yet, the relation between thinking and acting is, in principle, quite close. This somewhat complicated conception states, if I understand it correctly, the close relation of thinking to the world of reality and its multiform actions, as it has been pointed out above, and at the same time, the relative remoteness of the pictorial fashion of thinking from reality. At any events, the process of thinking is orientated towards the motor, acting, side of the personality.

H. Ellis, on the other hand, cites in his work a few older authors who stressed the tendency of the psyche to transform acoustic and optic impressions into motor images, and to connect them with motor associations. The concept of " high and deep sounds " originates in this tendency. Piderit is quoted as having stated (*Mimicry and Physiognomic, 1867*) that all our thoughts and feelings tend in a reflex-like manner towards the expressive motor side of life.[1] According to H. Ellis, this fact explains the tendency of dreams to dramatise feelings and other mental elements. The psychic condition is transformed into an active scene. I believe that there is much that is correct in both these theories ; in any case they illustrate the close relation existing between the waking

---

[1] Compare with this conception the statement of McDougall who considers the " felt " emotion as the subjective aspect of instinctual conation.

thinking process and the dream-experience, in their functional aspect. This might serve as a foundation to the thesis that both functions are akin with regard to their biological status. *Conscious thinking tends towards motor expression ; psychic experiencing occurring within the dream (during sleep) is an active, "motor" experience.*

(21) I should not like to probe too far into the field of purely speculative philosophy, and thus interrupt more than necessary the gradual exposition of the dream-problem proper. But it seems to me that the point of view just mentioned is worthy of a yet closer scrutiny ; it seems to lie on the path leading towards understanding of dream-symbolism, of the phenomenon of dramatisation and personification in dreams. The word which could most aptly and tersely express the physiological content of the whole somatic and psycho-affective process of life (not the philosophical meaning of life) is *movement.* The same expression, and the idea covered by it, represents metaphorically every feeling, particularly those projecting into awareness by reason of their strength or contrasting character. We speak of emotion, of being moved, and of " moving " motive forces. The external world is perceived by us, because it " stimulates " our senses, our mind, because it sets them *moving.* Any sensual and mental experiencing is the perception of something external or internal, by means of such inner movement of the psycho-nervous apparatus. *If, then, the " experiencing " mode of dreaming constitutes not simply a fortuitous property of this phenomenon, but on the contrary its very essence, purposely aimed at as such by nature ; if not only the dreaming in general, but also its particular, character as " experience ", and the special fashion of this experiencing, is part and parcel of dreaming ; then I fail to see how events of the " self " could be experienced more richly and abundantly, more aptly and completely than by the " moving " dramatisation and personification of the endopsychic tendencies and processes.* If we look upon the " experience " character of the dream as a factor of primary significance, of implying a meaning, then objectification and dramatisation, and widening of the mental elements by the way of symbolic substitution, appear as the only possible, as the most obvious mode, at the disposal of human psyche during sleep, by means of which the ego-experience can find its realisation on the broadest possible basis. The ego-feeling of waking life contains also the experiencing of one's own personality, as it finds itself set into its environment, and

implies an ego influenced by, and reacting to, the surrounding. The *formal similarity* between this waking ego-feeling and the mode of self-experiencing in the dream, appears obvious.

(22) After these more general introductory explanations, let us take up again the main thread of our discussions, and develop further the problem of the symbolic and transforming representation of mental elements, on the ground of the results arrived at by study of the organ-sensation dreams and of that of the "auto-symbolic" dream-images. Organically stimulated dreams show in all clearness that they deal with conditions of the dreamer's body, or rather, as it has been explained, with the dreamer's personality, as influenced by the physical process in question. Auto-symbolic representations of thoughts and mental conditions in general, as revealed in the hypnagogic experiences, show the same characteristics. Freud (in the chapter on Dream-work) attempted to separate this latter group of dreams from the dream-phenomenon proper, stating that the hypnagogic experiences described by Silberer constitute a contribution to the dream-formation by the act of *waking thinking*, and ought to be regarded in principle as pertaining to the group of *day-residues*. We, however, do not find it possible to see such a fundamental difference. And Freud himself admits in his *Introductory Lectures* [1] that " there are dreams which permit, besides the psycho-analytical interpretation proper, an ' *anagogic* interpretation ', pointing to the higher mental functions as contrasted with the instinctual tendencies. The majority of dreams, however, have to be excluded in this respect." This distinction of Freud's implies a difference in the way of looking upon dreams, and in principle his viewpoint is that of the *instinctive causation of dreams* (i.e., that the dream-stimulus and the aim of dreaming are respectively infantile drives and their striving towards hallucinatory wishfulfilment). For us such a distinction cannot be valid, because we interpret the dream-event in all its constituents and aspects, and therefore we do not have to ask from which sphere—whether the instinctive or other personality levels—the individual dream-motifs originate. The presence of the " functional ", anagogic elements in dream is, for anyone who looks for them, an obvious fact, and their recognition is indispensable for any kind of active psychotherapy.

Both groups of dreams, then, treat of the personality, its

[1] Ch. XV.

condition and its content, more precisely of parts of this psychic content. I find it hard to see how the extension of this fundamental character, so obvious in the two kinds of dream mentioned above, *to all dreams*, would meet any logical or factual difficulties. In the first place, many dreams treat quite openly the waking problems of the ego, deal with the dreamer's own wishes, hopes, sorrows and fears. In so far as other strange persons occur in the dream, and the events taking place in it, seem to deal with the fate and life of these others, it is easy enough to prove in a sufficient number of cases by the way of dream-associations, the close relation to the personal problems of the dreamer. For instance, someone dreamed :

> **28.** I pass a house ; in the yard I see my late teacher H. sitting on a chair. I call to him : " Are you still so nervous ? " He does not understand my question, and I remind him that twenty years ago, when he was in love with a red-haired girl, he became very nervous when she fell sick.

The associations to the manifest dream show that the dreamer is in love with a red-haired girl ; but he could only marry her if one of his relatives, whom he has to look after, did not exist. The bearing of the dream on to the dreamer's own, actual problem is thus quite clear. What he " *does not understand* " points to something which he *does not want to see* ; he has repressed the alternative wish : If the girl he loves died suddenly by accident, that would also solve the problem and make his craving for her disappear. . . .

Apart from this, we can and must assume that from a deeper psychological point of view, images of the external world, of external persons, cease, for the subconscious at least, to be pure " objects ", and they become constituents of the ego, i.e., they become *assimilated ego-parts*. A young woman loses her husband after a short but happy period of married life, and she has to marry again for the sake of her child. At the time she is making up her mind, she dreams :

> **29.** I am on a swing which is being pushed from both sides. I feel content and happy ; I believe that my late husband and my fiancé are pushing in mutual harmony the swing on which I am sitting.

It is clear that this dream treats of the two harmoniously combined constituent parts of her ego, and not of the two men taken objectively.

The assumption, according to which persons in a dream may represent qualities, principles and tendencies of the ego (interpretation on the subjective level of Jung), is in good accord with the psychological thesis mentioned above. When, on the other hand, persons occurring in the dream, by reason of the collected material, must be taken literally, and in their objectivity (cf. dream 11), we recognise this also as self-evident ; because our relations to the objectively real, external world are essentially also " psychic facts " ; and what we are in such cases dreaming of, are actually these our *relations and attitudes*. This fact too, therefore, fits into our thesis that the dreams deal essentially with the whole psychic life of the individual, with the content and condition of the ego. If, however, the dreams seem not to contain elements of this kind, in particular when the figures and events of the dream show no intelligible bearing upon the objective world, no connection with the real, waking life of the dreamer, then we may be certain that we are confronted with pictorial elements and symbols. *For the dream—I wish to stress this— deals with the attitudes and relations of the ego to itself and its environment, and only and fundamentally with the attitudes and relations of the ego.* This is in full agreement with the conditions existing in the organ-sensation dreams, which quite obviously have the conditions of the ego as their object and content.

It might be, of course, objected that the organic stimulus enters into the dream process only as an additional factor, that its influence is grafted upon the pre-existing dream-material ; that, therefore, all the conclusions drawn from such organ-sensation dreams are not valid, and the alleged unitary nature of all dreams is not proven beyond all doubt. But one has to realise that the other, " psychic " dreams are also reducible to stimuli, in this case to psychoaffective stimuli ; that these stimuli arise from the dreamer's own ego (when toxic, meteorological [1] or telepathic moments influence the dream-formation, they do so only through changing the

---

[1] A female patient who was treated because of psychogenic depressive conditions, dreamt regularly of dead persons and of graveyards during nights preceding a cloudy, rainy day. Obviously the changing atmospherical conditions always stimulated in her the same complex. " It is possible that one day we may see a closer relationship between the cosmic rays on the one hand, and hallucinatory experiences in psychotics and normal people, dreaming included, on the other hand. In the meantime, we need to know that such hallucinatory experiences chiefly affect people of a certain level of experience, for which analysis of the Freudian type may form the chief bridge." (Dr. D. S. Fairweather, in his work on Diathesis.)

state of the ego) ; that therefore the conditions are the same. We have no logical or objective reasons for assuming two or more different types of dream-formation (as " purely subjective " and " objective " dreams) ; and in fact such an assumption would contradict everything we know about the functioning of the organism in general. It would be as if the basic character of a secretion, produced by a gland, were not essentially the same (apart from certain quantitative and qualitative differences due to various special influences). Quite definitely, there is similarly only *one unitary dream-process*, in spite of the manifold and varied character of its individual elements, features, colouring, and the different sources of its material. As will be shown more fully in Chs. X and XI, this unitary dreaming-process serves the " metabolism of the various dream-stimuli ". The dream, however, arises from the ego and treats, in all its parts and forms, the relations and conditions of the dreamer's own personality. *All the persons, actions, localities occurring in the dream are either parts of the ego, or express relations and conditions of the ego.* This will be admitted by all students of the dream, whatever may be their particular point of view. *And thus the personification in the dream of parts of the ego could be shown as a definite result of our explanations and arguments so far ; and also the background of this process has been illuminated, within the limits of our present-day knowledge.*

(23) At this stage we want to consider the various other fields in which pictorial representation is employed and ask : What causes the use of metaphors and allegories in poetry ? What induces the cartoonist, the impressionistic and expressionistic painter, what induces the language of all times and nations to employ so abundantly the pictorial mode of expression ? (We speak of the " thread of an argument " ; a wave of passion ; a load taken off one's back ; a fruitful idea ; to be at large, etc.). Surely, it is the need, by creating something *new*, to give more emphasis to the thought, the idea, to the sentiment ; to give it a broader content, and to emphasise one particular side of the complex of ideas at the expense of another, to underline and to embellish. The content of the thought becomes enriched through the newly added associations which belong to the substitute-image, and its meaning is becoming shifted in the direction of this symbolising image. The new image is always transformed, not only in its appearance, but

first of all in its deeper content. For this reason I reject the idea that there could be a simple substitute-formation in the field of dream-symbolism (however, for purposes of practical psychotherapy, particularly when one has to convey an explanation, a solution to the patient, this way of substitute-interpretation is usually the only one possible). Indeed, especially in dream-symbolism, one must go far beyond such a simple conception. As pointed out above, it is certain that the *scs.* contains the corresponding elements of consciousness in a form which is different, and *in its essence transformed.* A different system has different contents. It will be agreed that every conscious element has its roots, its subterranean parts in the *scs*, but that not every subconscious element has a corresponding conscious counterpart. It follows automatically from this conception that the part pertaining to the *scs.* cannot be qualitatively the same as that of the conscious layer, the only difference being that the former is *not conscious.*[1] None, perhaps, will assume that the properties of the deep system are exhaustively characterised by saying that they are not conscious. According to Freud's conception, too, it is rather a question of a different energy-cathexis than that of a different topical condition. But it is very likely that there exists also an essential difference of quality, that distinguishes the conscious and subconscious or unconscious elements ; a difference more substantial than assumed by Freud in postulating that *the repressed unconscious element contains only the " object-idea ".*[2] When a drive or an ideational content has to undergo a " repression ", this means in fact its qualitative alteration. Otherwise the psychoenergetic significance of such a process would be unintelligible, and its required effect improbable. When an erotic complex has found a symptomatic expression in a globus hystericus, we cannot but assume that the substitute-idea implies a true qualitative change. It is surely not simply a question of a " deceived " psychic organisation which is ready to accept a substitute " label " instead of that which has been, which *had to be,* repressed. It is not only the affective element, the affective charge of the complex, which is changed, but also its genuine conceptual content, the kind and extent of its associative links. We may compare these conditions

---

[1] It would be true, however, to say that every subconscious element *is being perceived*, in so far as it remains effective on the psychosomatic unity, i.e., *it has surely its share in the total ego-feeling.*

[2] Cf. p. 13.

with the "isomerism" in chemistry, where two compounds, though identical in their percentage composition, present substantial differences in their chemical structure and properties. Or perhaps, more aptly, with two benzene-rings which differ only by one single side-chain group ; yet, this small structural change implies an entirely different character in chemical reactivity.

The case of repression has been mentioned only as an illustration, in order to show the capacity of the *scs.* to transform mental elements. This process of transformation is, however, an intrinsic property of the deep-psychic system in general, and its ample use in the process of repression is only *one* application of this faculty. As Bjerre aptly says in his work on dreams, repression is surely *not* the only transformation-function of the *scs.* The elimination of psychic residues which have become unnecessary to conscious life is a second example of this kind of function, which has little relation to the act of repression due to moral inhibitions. The thoroughgoing different character, the *otherness* of the subconscious elements, is thus proved and illustrated by various kinds of observation and different considerations and conclusions.

(24) We want to insert here some details regarding the essential difference obtaining between *conscious and unconscious modes of thinking.* The elements of conscious thinking are clearly delineated and formed, because our need for clear orientation in the sphere of living of the individual requires this. Only the awareness and the feeling of a certain constancy and clear limitation of our ideas, suggest to us in a convincing degree the existence of a sufficiently constant orientation. The elements representing the deposits of external impressions and perceptions are being transformed by the *scs.* ; they are no longer images of reality, no photographs of perceived things, but individually coloured parts of the *scs.*, which, in their compound totality, express the ego-condition, as it exists at any given moment ; this being contrasted with the *objective picture of the external world,* as contained within our conscious sphere of thought. (In my conception the subconscious element proper is even further remote from reality, than is the isolated "concrete idea",[1] postulated by Freud, which after all does express some objective relations.) Whilst the world-picture, as represented in the "objective thinking",

[1] Cf. Ch. I, p. 13.

remains in its basic structure constant, the total picture of our *inner condition* is liable to undergo a constant change, due to the continuous metamorphosis of the individual elements. Just as there is a metabolism of the physico-chemical constituents of our organism, there exist similarly a metabolic metamorphosis of our psychoaffective " stock ". *The changing dream-events, mirroring, indicating these events, give an idea of these important continuous intrapsychic processes.* Thus, they suggest the total " active condition " of the psyche ; not merely its content. And just as the " physical metabolism " carries out the task of guaranteeing the constancy of physiological events, so have the multiform events, occurring within the subconscious and unconscious spheres, the dreaming-process included, to effectuate the *psychoaffective homeostasis.* The essential difference between conscious and subconscious thinking modes may be expressed by saying, that the *intrapsychic processes in all their multiformity are being prevented from entering into consciousness, and thus the latter system is spared the shocks of a considerable change and inconstancy.* The *scs.* and the dream, therefore, constitute a world of their own, a world in which images of external reality *are* present, but in a state of a certain independence, belonging more to the *ego* than to the outer reality. The *world of dreams* shows its independence sufficiently by the irrational conditions obtaining in it, by the unreserved acceptance of objectively impossible situations, etc. For the world of the *scs.*, on the other hand, this independent character is a justified, self-evident assumption, made probable, first of all, through its close relation to the dream-world, to the neurotic manifestations, to the psychogen parapraxia (meaningful errors of action), etc.

All these theories and statements about the *scs.* are not meant to satisfy the philosophical need for absolute exactitude. They are meant to describe the point of view of the practising psychotherapist ; primarily, of course, they indicate the individual way of the author of looking at the problem. Their practical value lies in facilitating a better orientation in the world of dreams of our patients, an orientation about the minor yet continuous intrapsychic variations of the so-called analytic situation. The insight gained in this respect, should, however, not lead anyone to reveal too much of it to the patient. Gutheil once said rightly,[1] that most of

[1] Oral communication.

what the analyst gathers from the dreams, by reason of his skill in interpretation, is destined for his own orientation. Active psychotherapy, especially if supported considerably by intuitive dream-interpretation, implies a certain risk ; it is an *art*, and unless the case under treatment is a simple one, caused chiefly by a recent conflict, one can never be too cautious.

(25) We shall now resume the discussion of our central problem and proceed to the investigation of the symbolising processes in the dream. First, however, we have to summarise what has been established so far. The subconscious form of a psychic element differs from its conscious form. It is easy to see how elements which encounter some resistance in consciousness, and which, therefore, are predominantly or solely destined for the sphere of the *scs.*, show this differentiation in an increased degree. In so far as the dream-level contains subconscious and unconscious elements, it elaborates such, already transformed, elements of the deep layers. The pictorial, indirectly suggested representation of these elements in the dream is indicative of their " otherness ", of the fact that the corresponding element in the *scs.* which is the source of the respective dream-symbol, is essentially different from its conscious counterpart. This " otherness " of the sub-conscious elements implies, therefore, not necessarily its being "repressed " ; and accordingly, the symbolising and pictorial mode of the dream is by no means expressive in principle of a *disguising tendency*. When a mental element is subconscious, be it for reasons of repression, or because it is *per se* incapable of being consciously thought, this being due to its complicated and too abstract nature, then its pictorial representation appears even more natural and unavoidable. Indeed, it is rather astonishing to find, that certain elements of the dream appear in fact *not* symbolised, but in forms of waking thinking. As mentioned already, the dream-level is connected with both systems of thinking.[1] It is, furthermore, not always an unprohibited element, quite free of repression, which appears openly in the dream. Aggressive actions towards friends and relatives, expressing subconscious negative sentiments and attitudes ; sexual acts which are anathema to the conscious thought of the dreamer—these occur quite frequently in dreams, without any disguise.

[1] Ch: I, p. 24.

In the case of pollution-dreams, there is an obvious reason for this fact. The intensity of the libidinous stimulation reduces the level of sleep, and brings it close to that of waking ; thus, perhaps, also influencing the particular form of the dream ; hence the more overt representation. It is indeed possible, that anything in dream, which is *not* disguised and not represented in a transformed fashion, is really closer to the conscious system, constitutes in fact a content of this conscious system, though practically, it might be annulled for clear, conscious awareness. (Annulment is, according to Stekel, a process by means of which a certain complex of ideas, or the memory of a certain traumatic event, becomes as if encapsulated in a " detached layer " of the waking conscious-ness, but not really repressed into subconscious spheres. There is a knowledge of it, but no awareness, except in the half-conscious day-dreaming.)[1]

Perhaps it is for the same reason that aggressive tendencies appear in the dream occasionally openly represented. The quality of sleep becomes less deep, because of the intensity of the affective reaction, connected with such tendencies, and the direct dream-expression in such cases is a function of the " waking " system.

(26) I think, further, that we are not quite mistaken in stating, that the basic action of the dream, the essence of its " motor " happening, is less subject to the process of trans-formation, than the persons, their characters and their ten-dencies ; i.e., *the action of the dream less than the " object " and " quality " categories.* A dream-example will show what is meant by this law. The following was dreamt by a young man, during a conscious mental conflict he had :

> 30. I am standing somewhere, holding a long, pointed, tube-like thing, made of paper, which I push forwards, towards my girl-friend Lucy, who is standing there on an elevated place, far from me ; between us there is a ditch. She is surrounded by other girls. I stab in her direction, as if I had a lance in my hand. Thereupon she disappears ; I run after her in despair. Her face was earnest, full of reserve. Was it some kind of religious examination ?

The associations to this rather obscure tube-like apparatus point in three directions. First, it reminds the patient of a

---

[1] In the intensified annulment of the obsessional neurosis the respective content is debarred even from entering the dreams during sleep. Cf. Ch. XII, p. 229.

plaything, a kind of telescope, through which, at the age of 7, he had gazed upon the genitals of a little girl with whom he was playing. She died early. It was said at that time, that the doctor had to use a long puncture needle in order to remove the pus, and that this procedure caused her great pain. Secondly, he is reminded of a plaything belonging to a child (his cousin) whose guardian he is, at the wish of his own mother, a duty which makes it difficult for him to marry. Only if the child were dead would he be able to reach his girl-friend. At the present, then, she remains *beyond his reach*. Thirdly, he admits to some annoyance with her ; she does not make any financial contribution, which would make their marriage easier, although she is in a position to do so. He even thought once it might be better if *she* were no longer alive ; or else, if *she* broke off her friendship with him (in the dream she appeared as reserved as she once was when she really did suggest something of the kind).

The overdetermination of this mysterious object is quite obvious. In the main, we find three elements represented in it. (1) The telescope, which helps to assuage the pain of separation, by making it possible to reach the beloved person visually. (2) Added to this, is the feeling experienced in the dream of being able to touch the girl by means of this object and so to reach her concretely. (3) The doctor's pain-causing needle ; and, hinted at by the associations, an instrument for killing (suggested by reference to a lance in the manifest dream). The *stabbing movement* in the dream is clearly recognisable ; yet according to the detailed description by the dreamer, it resembled at the same time, the manner in which he used to throw out his arms when he wanted to kiss his friend. The features of both movements are essentially well preserved in the dream, as compared with the conditions of reality. *The object itself, however, is comparatively heavily disguised.* In its function as a weapon, as an instrument for causing pain, it is completely unrecognisable. The person at whom he stabs in the dream is his sweetheart. But according to the associations, and the analytical material available, the death-wish is felt strongest in relation to the child-cousin who stands in his way. This, then, would be a complete disguise ; perhaps it should be mentioned that he is in the habit of calling his girl-friend " child ". The dream, as a whole, might be said to contain the following thoughts : I want to reach her ; perhaps I could reach her soon if the child were not there. But another way of solving my problem would be if she were to disappear from my view altogether. I believe that she will always remain beyond my reach because too many questions of conscience are involved (religious examination). If one looked at this dream without any knowledge of the associations, one could hardly surmise some coherent meaning in it. But the movement of *stabbing*, of *reaching out*, would be recognisable with some imagination ; it has come into the dream structure without any great distortion. Here is another example :

> 31. A large playground. All the pupils move about merrily, with the exception of one, who comes slowly into the foreground, bent over his stick. He looks rather indistinct, perhaps thin, pale, lifeless.

This dream was reported by the same patient. With regard to the main figure in the dream, he added. " This used to be a fellow-pupil in the grammar school ; he limped. He was the son of a widow ; so am I. Mother and son were very devoted to each other. The boy was definitely stupid, but later on he had the good fortune to marry an intelligent, pretty girl, with a very sympathetic character. He was an official, and became very conceited and proud. He never was as pale and thin as in the dream ; in actual life he was always smiling."

This dream, too, fails in its manifest form to show any intelligible relation to the conflict of the present. Only *one* relation seems comparatively obvious : the inhibited motility, the lack of vivacity, in comparison to the other children who are playing around merrily. This, of course, symbolises the patient's *bound status*, which makes it difficult for him to marry. This represents a pictorial substitute image, but one which is still comparatively easily recognisable, i.e., not very much disguised. The person of the dreamer, whose tied, inhibited condition is represented, has totally fallen a victim to the process of substitute formation ; similarly his mental suffering is only hinted at in the obscurity, in the lack of vitality of the dream-figure, i.e., it is also in a considerable degree disguised by the process of pictorialisation. *The lack of motility, on the other hand, is expressed more openly.* One might say : the fundamental thematic action is transformed once, the person and his condition are *multiply disguised*. From the idea which represents the actual patient, we arrive at the substitute figure only through several associations : first, the element of marriage, then the element of advantageous marriage (he was stupid and a cripple, yet he married a pretty girl), thirdly, the fact that he was a fellow-pupil and also the son of a widow. It needed all these similarities together, to enable the dream-figure to substitute fully the dreamer's own person.   Similarly, the thinness and listlessness do not constitute a *direct* association to unhappiness ; yet it is true, in time one becomes depressed and thin if one does not reach one's goal in love.   Lack of nimbleness of the body, however, and lack of freedom in our actions, are closely related notions in the world of conscious thought (more direct substitution).

It is possible to demonstrate one aspect more in connection with these dreams.   At that time the patient was suffering from certain weaknesses of erection ; it was this that led him to ask for treatment.   It is easy to find a suggestion of this fact in both dreams.   In the first dream it is the pointed, tube-like thing which *fails* to touch the beloved directly (she vanishes) ; in the second dream it is the *crippled foot* which suggests the manifest symptom.   It is easy for the experienced analyst to recognise these two symbols ; but *only* because they are so well known and proven.   They are also logically explicable, of course.   But there is *no* obvious conceptual nearness between the paper tube or the crippled foot on one hand, and the erective difficulties on the other ; this also supports our above rule.[1]   But it illustrates more than that ; it also supports our fundamental thesis regarding the origin of pictorial substitute-representation, according to which such modification is based on the previous modification of the psychic element in the *scs.* The dream does not simply depict the fact of erective impotence ; nor does it represent the penis in its functional weakness.   That would be no more than copying the content of the conscious idea.   The dream is concerned rather with representing those complex relations, which give rise to the symptom ; it depicts rather the broader circumstances, existing at the deep psychic level, which are responsible for the manifest disturbance.   The whole complicated affair, with all its points and sources of conflict, is brought together in the dream and the supplementary associations, into a total picture of the

---

[1] What, in fact, *does* enable the substitution, is the common character of being " unfit for *action* ".

situation. As in the first dream, so also in the second (through the children at play) it is the *child* which is indicated as an important motif of the conflict. The dream-figure underlines this motif by the supplementary disclosure, that mother and son were dependent one on the other. In the interpretation, this means that his young cousin and his fate, are similarly closely connected with the freedom of action of my patient. Besides, he had to look after this child to fulfil the wishes of his own *mother* ; he does not want to cause her pain by neglecting his charge and endangering the child's welfare.

More interesting, because of its greater complexity, is the following dream. It deals with the historical present. In the heavy, fateful days when the war was coming nearer to us, a patient of mine was faced, like many parents, with the alternative of keeping his child in England, or sending him abroad. A friend warned him by letter not to do the latter without very careful consideration. On the other hand, he himself thought of going later to Canada, in order to resume his musical career which had been broken off. During all the time my patient had forgotten the existence of a family with whom he used to be on friendly terms, and who had emigrated there some ten years ago. The head of the family was carving out a successful business career for himself, and his children were following in his footsteps. The friend, who had now written to him, appears to my patient in his dream, together with one child of the Canadian family :

32. My friend tells me : " Imagine, last night Mr. N's little boy came to my bed, clad only in his underclothes. *He complained bitterly about his father ; it appeared that he really knew nothing of the violent acts of his father.* Then I meet Mr. Star ; as usual, he didn't look too well, but was good-tempered and modest, and recognised me."

Associations : " I really have not thought of the family N. for ten years. Mr. Star was my private tutor some 20 years ago ; he was a very conscientious, religious man. Once he refused to tell me something important ; I was too young to be trusted, he said. N's little boy has the same Christian name as I have. He was a quiet sort of boy, but turned out to be clever and industrious. As the youngest, he was very much beloved by his family. The word ' underclothes ' reminds me of Mr. N., his father, who once appeared among us thus incompletely attired, without showing any embarrassment. Then suddenly

I remember a story which deals with unscrupulous ambition ; in this story, too, *underclothes* occur. Then I think of the word ' sub-conscious ' (in German, the *sub*conscious being called *under*-conscious)."

My patient's friend and Mr. S. both warn him to be conscientious. But this can be inferred only from the associations. For, both these men, particularly the friend, thought in fact much of my patient's conscientiousness and ethical principles ; in actual life he was quite beyond their criticism, and the mere appearance of both persons in the dream would have, in fact, suggested, rather, friendship. Yet on the other hand, *the fact that a boy complains about his father, is by the manifest dream quite openly expressed.* It seems as if the dreamer's conscience, awakened during sleep, had identified itself with the interests of his child ; here, too, the child does not appear directly, but is represented by *another boy.* Yet it is again the same boy " who is ignorant of his father's violent actions ", and who has no part in them. It refers to the fact that my patient is convinced that his own happiness would also contribute to that of his wife and the child. He sees in the attempted *emigration of all of them* a definite risk, but a risk worth taking. *His conscious thoughts show no trace of the idea, that as a father he would be acting actually unscrupulously.* Thus the dream-figure of the child represents two tendencies *of his own Ego* (consider the identity of names !) : the sentimental tendency which looks at the hardships in the present, and advises him to spare his child the pain of parting, and to neglect the problem of his *own* musical career ; and another tendency, the result of realistic thought, which impels him, however, to take the risk because it is unavoidable, because this is a question involving the common fate, i.e., the future of the family. Both these tendencies and considerations, are conscious, and they form the " *fundamental action* " of the dream ; they constitute also the opposing poles of the conflict-situation. Both these " *motives* " *of his psyche appear almost undisguised in the dream.* All the *other* details point to the quality of conscientiousness, to his unawareness of his own egoism, and to his possible career which is his final aim. But all this is carried out rather pictorially, disguised and personified. (The various other points of analytical interest which were also ascertained, are left out in this interpretation.)

(27) The reader may feel the need for a theoretical account

of the causes for this differential intensity of transformation. We might put it somewhat like this ! *The dream in all its parts depicts the relations of the ego.* Now, even in conscious thought, there are much greater difficulties in the way of becoming conscious of our character, our tendencies, our body, than there are in the way of becoming conscious of our *actions*, while these are actually progressing. Even the image of a *thing* always becomes linked with the idea of its *function*. When we think of a tendency, we automatically continue our ideation and think of the execution of this tendency. Conscientiousness, and lack of conscientiousness, are ideas of which it is difficult to think, without picturing them to oneself in connection with some practical example, i.e., without associating them with some particular conscientious (or unconscientious) action. Where it is not a question of some special, concrete action, the respective ideas [1] may be supplemented by images of: protesting, complaining about somebody or excusing oneself. To complain about somebody, or to protest against the behaviour of somebody, implies *accusation* ; and this constitutes the "action" supplementary to the concept of being "unconscientious". To excuse oneself ("I do not know anything about it ", as in the dream above), represents, on the other hand, an " action " supplementary to the idea of " conscientiousness ".[2]

I admit that this attempt at explanation sounds rather schematic ; as we, however, do not want to dwell on this point, we have to leave it at that, while recognising the gaps of our explanation. Neither do we think our thesis sufficiently proved by the three examples quoted, to justify its general validity. The reader might have the impression at first, that it applied only to the instances selected, and to similar dream-images. That, however, is not the fact. The more he will focus his attention during his own analytical work on to the aspect suggested here, and the more he will try to see and to recognise the mechanisms described, the more he will realise and acknowledge the general validity of the law propounded here. Unfortunately, I do not know if a similar observation has been described by any other author ; it appears to me obvious and self-evident.

In any case, it will, for instance, prove as a basis for the intuitive, and at first rather surprising, type of dream-inter-

[1] i.e., " conscientious " and " not-conscientious ".

[2] Also, actions and movements of a different purpose are more similar than qualities and objects.

pretation which was introduced and propagated by Stekel, but which, in fact, he never developed theoretically and in a systematic, argumentative way. We are justified in interpreting the action, or actions, of the dream-event in a sense not very remote from the literal one ; we are thus in a position to surmise a good deal of the actual, historical life, and of the consciously concealed or unconsciously repressed thoughts of the analysed individual. Persons, things, qualities, however, will have to assume a widely different and " distant " meaning in the interpretation. Thus, for instance, one of Stekel's " rules " is, *that excreta, all kinds of secretion, as well as blood, urine, pus, and water, can stand for each other in the dream ; they can also stand for the soul, or for money.*[1] (According to primitive conceptions, excreta and secretions and the blood are bearers of the soul, of life-energy [2] ; and in the language of the people usurers are commonly called blood-suckers.) Such remote symbolic substitutions might easily be regarded as only fantastic suppositions by those who possess no special experience in this type of psychological research. Yet, experience shows, that such a bold " jump " into the fantastic often enables one to find meaning, actual significance in a dream ; a meaning, moreover, which is shown to be correct in the later course of treatment by the contributions of the patient. Yet, even so, the unriddling of the "object category" will always carry greater difficulties with it than the interpretation of the dream-action proper. The confirmations which associations afford us in this latter field (cf. the dreams quoted as illustrations) may encourage us to interpret dream events, at least in their functional aspects, i.e., as concerning the subconscious psychic attitude of the individual, *actively*, i.e., without having recourse to free associations ; and this particularly when seeking information about the day-to-day changes in the analytical situation. (Cf. Chs. V and IX.)

(28) Although this book is not devoted to the problem of special dream-interpretation, I propose to add two short examples which could be solved only by means of the above-mentioned symbolic equation. A man involved in a difficult love-conflict, which took great toll of his energy, wanted one day to distract his mind and he occupied himself by writing a long letter to a friend, who used to be at times rather trying. The night after writing this letter, he dreamt :

---

[1] *The Language of Dreams.*   [2] Cf. *Genesis*, Ch. ix, v. 4.

33. I see my friend ; he looks ill or angry. Then there is a question of something happening without costs (without pus ?).

Free associations of the dreamer : " A sister of the friend in question, is suffering from serious purulent abscesses, which endanger her life. For that reason he is now even more nervous than usual. Strange to say, he does not irritate me recently, as he used to do. I think of him in a kindly way, without feeling as I used to, that he is rather annoying. The thought of him is almost a relief for me in my terrible conflict." The interpretation follows directly from these supplements. *The friend does not use up my nervous energy, as usual* (it happens " without expenses " or " without pus " ; pus would here stand for blood, this in turn for the symbolic meaning of that word, i.e., energy). The dreamer relates, that after having this dream, he somehow felt better. *His endopsychic reconciliation with his friend caused this alleviation.*

The second dream is taken from a paper by Feldman (*Psych. Praxis*, 1931, 1, 3). A man of 42 falls a prey to impotence, when his wife is advised to avoid the dangers of pregnancy, because of tuberculosis of the lungs. He imposes a three-months' continence period on himself ; but during this time subconscious memories of his youth become active again. These deal with a period when he was suffering badly from *bronchitis*, which forced him to lie in bed for long weeks, and to look after himself carefully for several subsequent years. Thus his *continence* and his *potency-disturbance* both served the purpose of his supposed *self-protection*.[1] The following dream confirms this :

34. I have intercourse and discover that the spermatozoa look rather like my sputum when I was ill.

This dream is reducible to the above-mentioned " self-protection complex " ; spermatozoa and sputum both represent again the life-energy.

The logical intelligibility of the above-mentioned symbolic equation might be suggested by the following train of thought. We have seen that fundamentally the dream represents the ego and its parts and tendencies. *It is only natural that parts of the whole may take one another's place in the symbolic substitution ;*

---

[1] There is no need to point out to the trained physician that the alleged method of " self-protection " was only a neurotic fiction.

this in spite of the fact that, of course, the various bodily fluids and energies mentioned differ essentially. *Yet they are all parts and bearers of the real personality, therefore all suitable to become parts of a symbol-equation.*

The same applies to another symbol-equation of Stekel's, according to which all the orifices of the body (ear, mouth, navel, anus, vagina, urethra) *may* represent one another ; provided the dream-conditions call for such symbolisation. Similarly, the replacement of the genitals by the extremities and the nose, becomes intelligible, as well as the displacement-mechanism in dreams in general.   When the symptomatology of the parapathies (affect-conditioned neuroses) makes use of the same displacements and substitute-formations, it simply carries out in reality the conditions obtaining in the dream-consciousness.   (Cf. the chapter on " Archaic and Infantile Traits " for a similar consideration in a rather different context.)[1]   Of course, in these affect-conditioned neuroses, and often also in dream-symbolism (although there not so universally, and not as a fundamental dream character), we find that displacement aims at making the complex more tolerable, and it is an effect of repression.   But even Freud has stated that sexual symbols, although they *may* be used by the repressive function, do not originate from it.   We must extend this conception to all dream-mechanisms of pictorial, indirect representation.   The basic mechanism of all symbol-equations lies in the nature of " dream-thinking " ; I believe that we have proved this thesis with regard to above-mentioned substitute formations.   *In general all symbolic representations are based on the principle that images of the external world, of other persons, have become for the scs. parts of the ego, and so they are aptly suitable to represent tendencies of the ego.*   (Cf. footnote, p. 155.)

(29) It is clear that in this chapter we have considered and described the transformation-process, and the symbolism of the dream, in the broadest sense.   We have made no fundamental distinctions between contents of conscious thought, tendencies displaced into the sub-conscious, or finally, contents which had been repressed from consciousness into the *ucs.* or belong solely to the *ucs.*   The dream transforms everything that is not quite identical with the content of consciousness ; yet all that appears in the dream, is usually an element already transformed from some deeper level.   For this reason we have

[1] Page 182.

made no distinction in our expositions between contents of the *subconscious* and of the *unconscious* ; what purpose could there be for doing so ? We are interested in the *dream*, in the conditions and relations obtaining on this level ; everything that can be found *there*, simply *is* the dream. The object of our main interest has been the dream-*symbolism*, the process of *transformation* per se ; not the individual symbols. From this latter point of view, however, we *must* agree with Freud that there are constant symbols, i.e., that concepts of sexuality (genitals, coitus), of family relationships (parents, children), of being born, of living and dying, *do* find their expression in certain relatively constant symbols. This problem has been studied and discussed most thoroughly by Jones, who starts from the ground of classical psychoanalysis, i.e., from the concept of the absolute unconscious on the one hand, and the fundamental infantile complexes on the other. *Theoretically,* there is a certain amount of justification for making a distinction between those symbols which represent *un*conscious material of *this* type (and which elements are actually represented by means of the more constant symbols, established by Freud and his closer followers), and the other pictorial representations and inconstant symbols. But it is easy to see that this procedure is justified *only* from the viewpoint of that psychoanalysis, which looks upon the above-mentioned mechanisms of the *ucs.* as the basic mechanisms of every neurosis, and which in its therapeutic analysis always *tends to arrive there.* I believe that we are today hardly in a position to estimate correctly the general significance of these infantile complexes ; much preliminary work and unprejudiced investigation will be yet required before that will be possible. Their *universal existence* may be regarded as certain (the *constancy* of the respective symbols might be adduced as a certain degree of proof for this ; but for a different explanation, see Ch. VI, (2)) ; their *universal importance* for the neuroses must, however, appear dubious at the moment. It is known that the more independent, free-lance psychotherapists consider them only when they come into the picture quite openly ; yet the successes of these other analytical therapies, in the treatment of neuroses, are also facts which cannot be simply ignored. (Cf. Ch. VI.)

CHAPTER III

THE EXTENT OF TRANSFORMATION, REACTION DREAMS *

(30) HERE we want to resume the discussion of the so-called " functional phenomenon ", studied and described by Silberer.[1] The remarkable experiments carried out by this investigator —and confirmed by others—clearly show how conscious trains of thought, preceding sleep, are continued and, at the same time, pictorially transformed in the subsequent dream-images. The same phenomenon can be found with respect to various subjective conditions and feelings, existing in the individual immediately before going to bed. These also reappear, transformed pictorially, in the hypnagogic hallucinations and short dream-experiences of the first · minutes of sleep. (Cf. also Ch VII (3).) It seems but natural to assume that events of the same " functional category ", which are, however, more subconscious and unconscious than those mentioned, are also likely to be represented in the dream in *a symbolical fashion*. There is every reason to assume that the deep psychic layers are of an immeasurable richness and extension, and that subconscious events of this functional type are represented in the dream as much as is the case with the traces of instinctive processes, which latter, themselves, can remain similarly unconscious. Very largely, the dream is painted in concrete scenes, its events are mostly " material happenings " ; it is hardly possible *not* to reach the conclusion that *a large part of these, formally concrete, images depict in fact the functional elements and processes*. Just as the well-known symbols of classical psychoanalysis are alleged to give a pictorial expression to the more concreté events of sexuality, to libidinous conditions and relations in general, to the concepts of birth and death, to the relations of the individual to his parents and relatives ; so it is equally self-evident that the more complicated and abstract

---

* Continuation of Ch. II on Dream Symbolism.

[1] Cf. pp. 36–7 in the previous chapter. " *Functional phenomenon* " refers to mental states, tendencies, and also denotes conditions of the body and of its parts, as contrasted with " historical " material and elements related to the instinctive sphere proper. A detailed report and criticism on Silberer's work and his originally somewhat different use of the expression " functional " is to be found in a paper by E. Jones on " Symbolism ".

endopsychic events *also* take their due place in the dream-process, where they are transformed similarly into *symbols*. However, essentially, the whole process of dreaming is an "abstract" hallucinatory event, and the symbols representing concrete events actually cover the *psychic perception and elaboration* of these primarily concrete facts. Thus there is not, even in principle, a difference between the functional and material element of the psyche and of the dream. (Cf. also Ch. II, p. 60, Ch. X (2), and Ch. XII (14), which renders our above supposition even more logical.) It is clear, then, that the great abundance of functional processes, occurring at the deep psychic levels, are depicted in the dream exclusively in the form of substitute-images. Interpretations as : that the *stormy sea* depicts the dreamer's *world of emotion* ; the small, frail boat, sailing on the sea, represents the path of life ; the orchestra is an expression of inner harmony (or disharmony) ; darkness and clouds the symbols of many mysterious problems which engage the individual's mind ; and other similar equations, must be regarded as probable, as possible in principle at least.

It is remarkable that some individuals interpret often spontaneously such elements of their dreams in a functional sense, without having been encouraged and instructed to do so. In the conscious self-perception of such individuals their intrapsychic world appears more markedly, than is the case in the majority of people, in whom this broad sphere of intrapsychic activity occurs almost without any distinct awareness of it. I assume, then, that these two groups of people are different only in the *manner of perception* of their functional elements, but *not in the actual possession* of such a complex functional inner world. We know people whose emotional and subconscious world of thought is very complex and rich, but who have, however, not the faculty of clear self-perception of all this. The dreams of this type of person will, therefore, constitute a rich source for the investigator, though not so for the dreamer's own conscious realisation. Often, however, a complex inner life of the kind mentioned *is* accompanied by the faculty of sensing the symbolism existing in the dreams. The spontaneous interpretations, given by this latter type of individual, furnish further proof of the symbolising processes going on continuously in psychic depth, and particularly for those in the dream-formation. They are people whose conscious thinking is more influenced by this symbolising depth-process than is the case in others. They are, in this respect, comparable to the gifted investigator who may see and fully realise a fact that remains hidden from his unsuspecting fellow-humans, but which fact represents none the less a universally valid natural law.

(31) A young man, of undifferentiated mental structure, who was suffering from ejaculatio præcox and a mild obsessional neurosis, dreamt in the first week of treatment : [1]

> **35.** An air raid is on ; I try to hide in the doorway of a house. A motor-truck drives past, and I succeed in jumping into the house so quickly that the car, which rushes past very near to the house, does not graze me.

I asked him to associate, and he remembered that a *friend of his brother, who owned a motor-truck,* used to live in a house, similar to that shown in the dream. This friend became their enemy later, for nationalistic and political reasons. In connection with his flight and taking cover in the dream, he said : " *It is as if one man allows himself to be pushed aside on the battlefield of life by others who are more violent.*" It should be emphasised that this patient as yet had hardly been influenced by the knowledge of dream-interpretation, and showed no special talent for interpretation himself ; and that this was the only instance of a functional, symbolical interpretation which he produced. The confirmation of his interpretation was easily found by the associative allusion to the faithless, and later so very aggressive, friend of his brother ; but even more so by the mere mention of this brother. The latter had caused much bitterness to my patient, both because of his more active and striving nature, and also because he wanted to dominate him. In the days when he dreamt this dream, my patient did not talk about this brother ; indeed, he himself did not recognise that his spontaneous interpretation pointed in fact to the brother and to his attitude towards himself. He was enabled to interpret his dream aptly, *only* because his inferiority feeling, which he actually experienced and suffered, was too intense to be overlooked by him. This constant feeling of inferiority has coloured his whole thinking, and influenced, therefore, the above association. What he even less recognised, because it was quite foreign to him up till then, was this : his parents

[1] Cf. Ch. XII, p. 221.

had always warned him not to become entangled with girls, and advised him even to put off marriage because of the obligations which such a state would impose. His parents, of course, led the usual sexual life and he, up to the age of 25, eavesdropped on their sexual actions, whereupon he experienced full satisfaction. He never admitted being annoyed with his parents for this system of " double standard ", although this would have been the most natural reaction. But during the same period as the dream mentioned above occurred, he dreamt also :

36. The girl-friend of my brother is " petting " with her boss. This makes me very angry.

He admits, when questioned, that the boss in the dream resembles his own *father* in appearance and even in age. His interpretation of being pushed aside, originates *also* (and if looked upon analytically, even mainly) from this source. It is interesting to add that the patient himself did not refer his interpretation of being pushed aside to the members of the family at all, but to the world at large. This may serve as an indication that the average dreamer, who has not been trained in analysis, and who does not belong to the category of the above-mentioned " philosophically natured " people, is not in the position to recognise mental contents, if they are expressed in the language of the dream, unless these thoughts represent concepts of which he is wholly, and intensely enough, conscious.

Earlier on, the same patient had dreamed :

37. I am driving to a neighbouring town where my brother's girl-friend lives. I encounter spies.

I suggested the interpretation, that he felt himself in all his actions watched and interfered with by his moralising parents. This interpretation he accepted very readily ; even much later he often remarked how correct he had felt this idea of the analyst. Here, too, we are dealing with an intensely and constantly experienced content of his thinking and feeling. Hence the ready acceptance of my interpretation. Clearly the position is, the more repressed, the more abstract, and " unthinkable " or " not easily thinkable " material, a certain psychic complex contains, the more symbolically transformed will it reappear in the dream. This is essentially what we suggested earlier, as the fundamental law of symbolism : that it is primarily the intrinsic difference between the subconscious and the corresponding conscious element, which gives rise to the symbolic and figurative mode of expression ; that reversely everything which appears symbolically in the dream-image, *is* different in its subconscious root, as compared with the corresponding conscious part.   Thus, in the last-mentioned example the spies express the deep-seated inner inhibitions, which have been established in his psyche as a consequence of parental guidance, and which have become a stabilised constituent of his mental make-up.   Even the little we have said, may give some idea of the wide ramifications of this particular complex of the patient.

A possible alternative formulation of the dream-theme might have been : " My parents come into the room when I am going to have intercourse " ; but this would and could express barely even a fraction of the total pathogenic inhibiting complex ; and thus this whole complex has to be depicted quite differently by the dream-image.   In a good many cases, we are enabled to gain some insight into the various ramifications of the complex in question, because the choice of the "symbol", and the various parts of the dream, lead in various directions pertaining to the complex in question.

Such is the case in the first-mentioned dream of this patient (No. 35), where the associations led first to his homeland, then to the topic of the unreliable friend, i.e.; to the bipolarity of human relations ; and lastly to the tyrannical brother.   I may add that after a few minutes of producing associations, the dreamer said that he did not like this particular dream, and that he was thinking constantly of the other dream, about the girl and her employer (No. 36).   In other words, this second dream became *a free association to the first,* which again had opened up the way to the parent-complex.   All these strands are woven together into a unity which explains his sexual inferiority-complex, and also the dream-experience of being pressed against the wall ; they are the factors which gave content to his inferiority-complex in general.

Here is the dream of a woman patient, who came for treatment because of agoraphobia and general anxiety :

> 38.   I am in a dark room, I see people there ; many children and also a peculiar wall.   I do not feel very happy.

At the time when this dream took place, the agoraphobia

for weeks had been improving to a considerable degree; similarly her pleasure in life. She was a 50-year-old woman, who, during her 25 years of marriage, had suffered from vaginismus, and from lack of libido. Her husband, also 50 years old, showed little desire now to keep pace with her. He lacked all interest, was always tired, and had no understanding of the finer, delicate aspects of life. The pitiable woman was faced with a new, for her, fully conscious conflict : she had no opportunity of being mentally healthy and normal. Her anxiety states recurred in a weakened form, whenever the husband refused to understand her wistful suggestions and tiredly went to sleep. When I asked her to produce free associations, she showed at first obvious resistance. She maintained she had nothing to say to the dream, and had never seen a wall of that kind. Yet, when I insisted, she recollected the wall of the mental home where two of her brothers were detained with schizophrenia. This fact, as well as her continuous fear of going mad herself, was one important source of her disturbances. I explained to her that at her age such fears were groundless, since the illness of her brothers was of a kind that never occurs in people of her age. When pressed for further associations, she remembered the wall of another hospital where she had been a patient as a child, and where she had seen a dead body for the first time in her life. Her stay in this hospital was associated also with a " gain through illness " [1] ; it was the first and the only period of her life that she, the child of poor parents, was made a fuss of, was praised, and given presents. She had been sorry at that time to have to return home. Both these trains of thought show relation to her being ill at present. Her resistance, her reluctance to continue associating, was plainly visible on her face. Then suddenly she cried : " But all this doesn't mean anything. That sinister wall represents my unapproachable husband. He is stupid and he will never be different. *There will always be a wall between us.*"

We can but fully agree with this interpretation. An unfortunate woman who is on the road back to health, and who experiences this return to health by the heightened urge of her libido, of her interest in her husband, has to recognise that for her there is " no further progress on this road ", that there looms before her an unsurmountable wall, barring the way

[1] Comparable with the pleasure-reward of neurosis.

to the desired freedom.   The dark, gloomy memories of her childhood, upon which she had been fixated, threatened to become again active, pathogenous complexes.   The darkness, the peculiar wall, symbolise the inhibiting, health-menacing elements, as well as the realisation of being powerless, of being unable to fight the real sources of her illness with any success. For the *consciousness* of the dreamer, however, the only understandable factor is the unfriendly rôle of the husband, but not the total difficult condition of the psyche, with all its hereditary and   acquired   pathological   complexes.   Consequently,   we must say that the interpretation of the patient was correct, though not complete.   What she wanted, was real, concrete happiness, not further theoretical submersion in the depths of analysis.   The dark room and the wall, are also expressions of her resistance against further analysis.

In this case, as well as in a few others, it became clear to me that the ready recognition by the patient of the functional symbolic meaning, represents some kind of *resistance*.[1]   The mental mechanism of such individuals makes it easier to bear the distressing contents, by transforming historical memories into pure psychological experiences.   This process is essentially analogous to Freud's " screen-memories ", where one repressed event is represented in consciousness by another, apparently unsignificant.   For people of this type, thinking along symbolic and functional lines, is a sort of flight from the distressing reality.   By looking always for the psychological and functional higher aspect in the events of life and in the life of dreams, they annul to a certain extent the force of concrete external reality in general, and thus implicitly the reality of their own oppressing life-traumas.   When under analysis they see and understand so readily the functional aspect of their dreams, they employ, in fact, for purposes of disguise and resistance, a mental mechanism which they possess habitually, and which is a special mode of their psyche to strengthen their general repressions.

(32)   Our knowledge of dream symbolism, and the confidence in our attempts at interpretation, can be furthered and strengthened by investigation of the *closer relation obtaining between the manifest dream and the latent dream elements, as discovered by the process of associating*.   Examples may serve to make this relation

---

[1] I have found a somewhat similar remark in the paper by Jones on " Symbolism ".

clear. It is necessary in practice to spare no pains when searching for the conscious sources of the individual dream-element. If this is done, one is enabled, partly at least, to appreciate the extent of the symbolic transformation, which is the intrinsic property of the dream-work. A colleague, in training-analysis, reports the following dream :

> **39.** The dream takes place in a lecture theatre. The dictator points to, or says something. I am bored, and with several others I creep away. But I think better of it, and I return to the hall, because otherwise the tyrannical lecturer might notice that I am no longer in my accustomed place. But then I find myself on the other side of the hall, and who knows if he will take notice of my being there ?

Here are the detailed associations regarding the source of the dream-elements : " The whole place reminds me of the great hall of a university which I once visited in order to be present at the graduation of a colleague of mine who was at the same time my patient. I didn't like it much there, most of the people were loud and *chauvinistic*. Also the brothers of my young colleague took only scant notice of my presence, although they probably knew that I had cured him of a serious disease. The dictator reminds me of a political personality of the present ; and at the same time, I am reminded of one of my teachers who, in spite of certain good qualities, was guided mostly by prejudice and desire to rule over *others*, and who, through his lectures, had spread more hatred than human science. I also think of a woman, herself a doctor, at whose house I was boarder at the time of the dream and who, though not void of some goodwill, was a paranoid and autistic person and restricted the private life of all who lived with her. To myself I used to call her the worst *tyrant* I had ever met. The father of the above-mentioned patient-colleague was similarly a *pathological character and a petty tyrant*. Before going to sleep, I had thought of a letter which I had sent abroad, and which might undeservedly cause me some embarrassment. I considered making amends for my mistake, but remembered that the addressee, who was terribly *obstinate*, would not carry out my wishes, and that all my endeavours would be in vain. This man, too, who is a good friend of mine, had been annoying me considerably in the recent past, and I wondered if he was worthy of my attachment and consideration. I should have liked to go to see an amusing film, *The Tyrant of the House*, but

I did not go for the sake of a fellow-boarder, who, however, did not deserve such considerations on my part. Yet, I wanted to prevent him from becoming envious. Before going to sleep, I also thought of how useless and hopeless it is to try to convince paranoid people by logical arguments and by kindness ; their delusions and prejudices do not permit of any insight on their part. But one has to do one's best to *prevent further trouble*."

The dreamer continued : " Having recorded these my associations, I feel clearly that the dream (on its *actual level*, i.e., with regard to experiences of the present) constitutes a reaction to my disagreeable environment ; giving at the same time expression to my fear because of the letter (possible troubles with authorities), and to my anger because of my friend's obstinacy. In order to carry on at all, I have to continue to bear my present stifling environment ; and I am also unable to react in the proper manner to the unjustified behaviour of my obstinate friend. I am, therefore, really under the heel of *dictatorial, tyrannical influences*, and I must relinquish every plan of escape, in order not to be even worse off than I am. In the dream this latter thought is suggested by my contrite return ; and the poor gain from my surrender in my actual life, is represented in the dream by the anxiety whether the dictator will really notice and appreciate my presence.

" Apart from this particular conflict, I was faced also with another question which required a quick decision. I had the opportunity of taking over a surgery, but in doing so I should lose all hope of continuing my analytical profession which I started only recently and also my hobby for writing. I should be tired in the evening, desirous only of rest, and I should have to give up all contact with my friends, particularly with that mentioned above because the job I had been offered would take me far away from my present residence. I am very fond of surgery and of clinical medicine, but not fond enough to give up everything else for it. Also I was rather afraid to be second in authority to the doctor whose surgery I was supposed to do, and to be a stranger in the surroundings where I had to live ; under such circumstances any accident or failure might have grave consequences. This concern, too, is alluded to in the dream, by the loud, chauvinistic people, by the Jingoish professor, and by my leaving the hall. The evening before this dream, I had spoken about the difficulties which would await a doctor of a foreign nationality, and only in incomplete knowledge of the local habits. I had spoken so in the presence of my landlady, whose autistic and very nationalistic attitude I wanted to probe. However, in the main, the dream showed *only me, facing in helpless concern my two main recent problems.*"

The following dream of the same dreamer is quite interesting, showing a different sort of reaction to a different kind of conduct on the part of the same paranoid landlady. As for previous history, it should be mentioned that the dreamer, the evening before, had fallen suddenly ill and had to lie down for a few minutes. The landlady was terrified and looked after him with great sympathy. This was only partially agreeable to him ; he would have to feel grateful to her for her services. Carrying such ambivalent feelings around with him, however, would certainly be an additional burden for his troubled psyche. This was his dream :

> **40.** A girl speaks to me about some *old gentleman* who lives in the neighbourhood. He is supposed to have done me some service ; he has used his influence in order to get me a post with the Council. *I did not want the post particularly ;* also I did not like the old gentleman very much, and hated the idea of owing him a debt of gratitude. I knew, however, that I *had* to thank him cordially.

The basic action of the dream is so clearly related to the events of the evening before, that no special explanation of this fact is required. What should be pointed out, however, is a substitution of the landlady by some unknown old gentleman ; and similarly the original cause for the disagreeable gratitude by the post with the Council. The dreamer continued : " In connection with the old man I remember a stern but not unsympathetic person whom I used to know as a child, and who was very *unkind* to me on one occasion. I remember having thought of his ripe old age and probably imminent death. This points to the theme of *revenge* against the landlady. As regards the locality, it reminds me of the garden of a modern hospital where I did surgery and at the same time of the lawn in a *cemetery.* In connection with the post it should be pointed out that at the time of this dream (several weeks before the previous one was dreamt), I had to consider my return to organic medicine. In the dream my feelings with regard to this return do not seem quite decided, which is

in good agreement with my conscious thoughts and considerations which I had at that time on this subject. Among other
things I was afraid, for hygienic reasons, of becoming a resi-
dential doctor in an overcrowded sanatorium at a time when
there was in the country an influenza epidemic, and when the
work might be extremely heavy." The allusions to hospital
and churchyard (danger of death), in the associations, are
intelligible also from this latter point of view.

(33) For the following example, and the whole associated
material, I am indebted to another colleague of mine who
suffered from palpitations, slight depressions and insomnia,
and who had a fairly sound theoretical knowledge of psychoanalysis. The preceding events, as far as they are relevant
to the dream, are as follows :

" I am now living in the same house as a woman relative who
has been divorced from her husband. At times she tries to be
very kind to me, but this is very annoying to me because she
is of a neurotic selfish type, and consequently often very disagreeable. Her relatives are also *pathological* individuals and
at every family meeting there are strongly neurotic scenes.
One of these scenes took place on the evening before the dream.
I was sorry for them ; but at the same time I felt some sort of
malicious joy, saying to myself : My selfish and funny relative
annoys me with her groundless accusations ; now in turn she
has become the victim of similar ' fictions ' of her brother.
She was very hurt, because I quietened her down only after
a fashion, without any great show of true sympathy ; she felt
I did not take her quite seriously. Originally, she developed
an intense transference-affect towards me ; but after the
manner of neurotic people, this liking for me was soon mingled
with distrust and accusations. In the last few weeks I had
tried to restrict talking to her and if I did speak, only superficially. I used to listen silently and without overt interest,
especially when I feared that her complex of selfishness might
be touched and stirred up."

41. My mother and a poorly dressed tall man are standing
near the table. He is cutting bread for dinner, and says,
directing his remark at me, that only blue flour, type 4, ought
to be used for reason of economy. I am annoyed, place myself in front of both and make a long speech, flowery and full
of allusions against the man. I remember only saying, that
a stranger is hardly in a position to look into the soul of others ;
and that a man into whose soul the others cannot see, just

because he has no soul at all, has no right to give orders to me.[1] The man listens quietly and proudly ; then he gets up and runs away. My mother gets up sadly, and goes to the window behind the curtain. I am afraid she might commit suicide ; I follow her, but she is annoyed with me, takes an umbrella and stabs my heart in revenge for the insult which I have offered her visitor.

" Dream sources which belong obviously to the manifest content and which do not require deeper going interpretation, are the following : the *tall* man, *poorly dressed*, who listens *quietly* and *proudly*, reminds me of *my* cautious silence, enforced by the difficult surroundings in which I live. The *poor clothes* fit in, too, because I had thought it was only my bad financial position which compelled me to stay in this household. The day before I had said to a very pleasant gentleman of my acquaintance—*tall*, elegant, *always quiet*, and not much given to talking—that I had to postpone a certain visit because, for the sake of preserving my only good suit, I decided not to wear it for a certain time. The man in the dream has a *beard* which is *turning grey* ; this reminds me of my *father*, who in his later life used to have a *beard* which was similarly grey. I believe he often *kept quiet* when my mother had nervous outbursts. But the dream-figure itself is a completely novel formation of the dream-work ; I cannot reduce it as a whole to anything known. Eyes and mouth could be derived perhaps from a teacher, whom as a child I used to adore, but whose severity I condemned. This man was remotely related to my mother, who had often praised him in comparison to my father, who was also a teacher, but who never inspired as much respect as the other. With some exaggeration it might be said that my mother adored this teacher. The *blue bread* and the *flour, type 4*, led to the following associations : *blue-green mildew on bread* during the 1914–18 war ; I was at that time a pupil of the just-mentioned stern relative of my mother. I was forced at that time to economise. When I was young we at home used to make do with *washing-blue*, instead of a different material which was not obtainable in war-time. Further, I am reminded of a *green-blue poisonous substance* which a school friend used to play with, in his small chemical laboratory, while we children watched with awe and envy. The *blue* suddenly recalls a part of another dream which I had the same night, where I make an injection and the patient starts

---

[1] Resistance against the analysis.

bleeding—subcutaneous congestion of blood turns *blue*. My relative cut her finger the day before, but in fact I did not see the wound. Type 4 reminds me that at school our work used to be marked by numbers, and in Czechoslovakia 4 or 5 signified bad scores. I am very abstemious in food, but in the household in which I live, everything appears on the table in plenty, except bread. My relative is always praising herself for all the care she takes of me ; the evening before, she told her father-in-law that she did more than necessary for everyone, myself included. This annoyed me and I determined to be even more *taciturn* than before. Flour, I certainly have not spoken or thought about recently. My mother was very conservative and self-sacrificing, but discontented in her marriage, and she often hysterically reproached my father. But it is quite inconceivable that she should have had even a platonic friend. She was fixated upon *me*, and she used to become *annoyed* when I did not seem to be sufficiently loving. In my feeling I relate the figure of my mother in the dream to my neurotic relative. The age would be just about right. So would the affection for me which, however, in this case, is strongly disguised ; the dream apparently re-awakens the memory of the neurotic attitude of my mother. I am also convinced that my relative turns her anger against me, because she is jealous and feels rejected. . . ."

It is quite clear that the dreamer himself has tried to find a mother-image in the relative, but that this transference was rendered unsuccessful by her neurosis ; consequently he is forced to restrain himself artificially, to " economise " not only with regard to words, but also with regard to his feelings towards her. He takes revenge on his relative for this feeling of disappointment, by destroying in her, too, every hope she may have cherished in connection with him. This second, suffering ego, *disappointed and disappointing*, is represented by the tall man. (We shall leave out of account the allusion to the dreamer's own father, and to his Œdipus complex, of which he was quite conscious.)

For the symbolic interpretation we get the following equations or substitute-formations. The *economical use of flour* points decidedly to the restrictions, which were forced on the patient through the selfish neurosis of his relative ; he must be restrained in word and emotion. The *blue flour* signifies the *distressed condition*, materially, and particularly mentally, in which he finds himself. At the same time, it signifies *poison and revenge* against the relative. The *grey beard* of the man in the dream, and his *poor clothes*, signify the *distressed condition* of the dreamer *as a man*—his jealous relative prevents any friendship with women ; thus making him into an *old man* before his time. *The umbrella* points to a complicated event, connected with the hysteria of the patient's mother, going right back to his earliest youth. No other associations were forthcoming in connection with this dream-element. The final scene of the dream cannot be interpreted otherwise than that the mother and her neurotic behaviour had from the very first hurt the patient's heart (psychically and organically). (The " classical psychoanalyst " would here invoke the " phallic mother ".[1]) *Heart* represents perhaps the genitals too (displacement from below upwards) ; the dreamer thought at times that he would lose prematurely his sexual fitness, in consequence of his worries in the past and present.

One part of the substitute-representations is quite close to conscious thought and usage ; " economising " as an expression of need and restriction ; " grey beard " as allusions to age and inhibited manliness ; " poor clothing " as a symbol of psychic distress, are logically quite understandable. Other substitutions, such as the allusion to the " inferiority of the bread " by means of the blue colour, and also to the blood and poison by the same element, appear rather remote and logically far-fetched. The " umbrella ", which stands for, or replaces a whole complex, a dramatic period of the individual's life history, is an instance of a kind of substitute-formation which is considerably different from the usual conception of " symbol " ; although fundamentally, of course, this kind of substitute-formation and the usual symbolism lie along the same line. This example shows clearly that the relation, the closeness of the substitute-image to the concept for which it is substituted, or the complex which it alludes to, may be of a various degree and kind. This difference is even true of various parts of the same dream ; and all the more so of the dreams produced by different individuals. Thus we find that the substitute-formations of some people can be interpreted easily, whilst those of others only with considerable difficulty. In such cases, the path of association, leading from the symbol to the original concept or complex, is longer or

[1] Freud : *New Introductory Lectures.*

more roundabout, than with the former group of dreamer.   In some cases it might even happen that the substitute-formations run essentially along purely individual paths as, for instance, in the case of the umbrella in the last dream which, in fact, covered a certain period of life, and stood at the same time for a complex of ideas connected with the dreamer's mother.

I should like to mention at this juncture, that some individuals when asked to produce associations to a certain element, stated by Freud to belong to the sexual class, do this in a clear and straightforward way, illustrating obviously the respective equation.

An acquaintance of mine who once spoke about her fright when coming across a mouse, was asked by her husband to produce free associations to the element " mouse ".   She enumerated without hesitation, and totally ignorant of Freud's symbolism, the following words : Mouse, mousehole, ran into it, skirt, aeroplane, flying.   The respective symbolical meanings are too well known to need special explanation.   Freud, however, pointed out that as a rule his sexual symbols are not followed by free associations pertaining to them, since the associated affect of inhibition does not permit of this easily, and such symbols have to be directly interpreted.

An important position among the purely individually conditioned symbols, is taken by the *periodically returning, stereotyped dreams and dream motifs* in the dream series of one and the same individual.   The psychoanalyst suspects rightly that the dream motif which is being repeated with such persistence, contains important hints of deep-rooted complexes, which have to be therapeutically tackled.   The inexperienced analyst will find that sometimes his endeavour to unearth the origin of these dream-motifs is attended by therapeutical success ; but that in other cases, even the most beautiful and apparently fitting interpretation yields no practical result.

I have found that these motifs had undergone a change in significance as time went on ; that during the course of treatment they no longer, not altogether or not mainly, represent and suggest *that* material, from which the constituents of the image or of the motif originated.   One gains the impression that the frequent appearance of such recurrent motifs renders therapeutic efforts more difficult, because we are then dealing with a progressive secondary formation, i.e., a complex which is still connected with the primary content of the image in question, but has been considerably broadened, by further subconscious contents, which latter have hardly any connection with the original form of the dream-motif.[1]

In one of my cases there appeared a *baby* in almost every second dream. The feeling-quality of these dreams was sometimes positive, sometimes negative, a fact which by itself indicates the differential valuation of that dream-motif. It was noticeable that these " baby-dreams " recurred regularly, whenever there was an obvious analytic resistance, and whenever the patient thought that she had some reason to feel a grudge against me, or whenever she felt depressed because of certain domestic difficulties, though they had ceased to appear for several days. It was clear, therefore, that in this case—and similar observations showed the same—the " baby-dream " indicated various items related to the patient's illness and treatment. It was possible in this case to throw a good deal of light on the origin of the recurrent motif. The birth of a younger sister, when my patient was six years old, caused her much concern, and even after she had grown up, she thought that she had lost, through this sister, the love of her much admired father. She remembered also that the first traces of her present obsessional symptom (she had the feeling that things were not even, and not symmetrical) appeared after the birth of the sister. It is obvious that the " baby-motive " has become an *individual mode* of expressing all her neurotic mental contents and reactions,[2] and an indestructible part of her psychic mechanism of expression.

(34) A poor nurse who had not received her salary for some time, and had been put off with lies and promises by the *matron* of the nursing home, dreamt during the night, after her last abortive attempt to get her money :

> 42. I am having a heavy *quarrel with my mother* ; I want to go to Shanghai, but my mother refuses to buy me the three white frocks which I want to have for the trip.

The dreamer never had wanted to go to Shanghai ; but once she attempted, though without success, to send *money* to a friend there. This connects the Shanghai motif to the *money* motif, and may convince those who doubt that the dream, which, after all, does *not* show any direct reference to the withheld salary, is really a *reactive formation* to the annoying experience. In connection with the mother, the dreamer, who

[1] Cf. Ch. XII (8), (10).   [2] Cf. Ch. VI (6).

always spoke about her father very enthusiastically, said : " My mother was always very busy, she ran a home for children, and so my father was always closer to me." Psychologically, then, her mother, in fact, similarly deprived her of something, viz., time and personal attention. This makes it easy to see how the present disagreeable position stimulated a mother-dream. The close connection becomes even more obvious when it is remembered that it was a *matron* who owed her something, i.e., a mother in a different sense.

Now we shall investigate whether we are dealing here merely with a substitution of the person in question, or with a more extensive substitution of the whole content ; i.e., whether the dream was really aimed at the matron, and found its manifest expression through the mother-image ; or whether it was aimed at the true mother, and the reproach against her mother was released from the depth of her psyche by the actual event of the day. The psychotherapist who is interested only in the practical aspect, will simply assume that we are dealing with a *condensation* of conscious, recent factors and of co-conscious, more chronic factors. The more orthodox psychoanalyst will say that the actual day-event has released the infantile Electra complex (hatred of the mother in this case). If taken from a practical viewpoint, then *both are surely right in their working hypotheses.* I believe, however, that some additional considerations will serve to deepen the insight even of those who are concerned chiefly with the practical side. For several days I was a witness of the annoyance of the poor nurse, and can testify with certainty that *this affect by itself* was quite sufficient to engage her psychic apparatus and the world of her dreams. There is no doubt that the dream cited, refers to the actual event of the day before. I feel tempted to assume that the annoyance and her contempt for the selfish matron, had brought about her annulment in the dream ; the dream says roughly : *If I have to give rise to so much emotion, and if I have to suffer all this, then I should prefer it to be due to my mother, for whom I feel deep affection as well as hatred. . . .* At the same time, the recent event helps to abreact, at least partially, the chronic sentiment felt towards her mother. Also, it often happens in ordinary life, that despair over some actual misfortune makes one more conscious of all the other disagreeable things one has additionally to endure. It is all the more difficult to bear the present burden, the heavier are the accumulated burdens originating in the past. In summary, we may say that the actual event is transformed into a mother-scene because the " extensive " and " personally more import-ant ", includes the " lesser " and " less important ", of the same group of feelings ; and because, as suggested above, the mother-conflict was still easier to be borne since it contains, however, a partial pleasure (ambivalence). *This factor makes it psychobiologically easier, to abreact the recent conflict in the mother-disguise. Thus, the substitution shows both, meaning (extension of the problem), and biological purpose (facilitation of abreaction).*

A similar mechanism lies at the basis of the dream-work, which, as described already, projects one's own suffering on to others, which displaces the troubles of the *ego* to others. These are *mechanisms of relief, attempts at elimination, possessing a quite definite biological significance.*[1]

If these my suggestions—which essentially corroborate and supplement the more usual interpretations as mentioned first —are correct, then they enable us to explain the diverse manner in which the latent dream-material is transformed into the manifest dream. *It is psychobiological necessities* which deter-mine the extent of substitution, and which cause the difference between the unconscious form of the mental contents and their conscious counterparts. The event to which the dream changes and transforms the original material depends, partly, on the structure of the personality, and partly on the recent state of the psychic apparatus ; this condition of actuality in its turn represents the result of other psychosomatic events, not least among which are the more or less disturbing physio-logical and psychological stimuli, which influence, at the moment they prevail, the psychic apparatus, dreaming included. It is for this reason that psychoanalytical interpretation of dreams will always remain an art, rather dependent upon sudden flashes of insight, and never a purely mechanical process of mere logical deductions. The " intermediary pro-ducts " of psychic happenings are never as uniform and as constant as those of organic metabolism ; this implies the fact that the content and meaning of any given dream-element is a variable factor.

The above dream and its total background, illustrates very well the phenomenon of the " *affect-displacement* ", which Freud has emphasised so strongly. " The affect appears completely

[1] Cf. Ch. II (12), (13), (14).

divorced from the idea-content to which it belongs, and is deposited elsewhere within the dream." [1]   Such displacement of affect takes place, even more markedly and intensely, in the cases of certain phobias and obsessions where a substitute idea has taken possession of the respective affect.   *Reaction-dreams such as the last cited ones, show this displacing phenomenon in statu nascendi (during their origin) like an experiment.*   We assume, of course, here as elsewhere too, quite non-dogmatically that the actual situation has really enriched the dream-content and dream-affect to a substantial degree, and that, therefore, the dream actually gives expression *also* to the recent situation.

(35) Here follows another example.   First the preceding event.   A music teacher treated one of his pupils in a very impersonal matter of fact manner.   He noticed that this pupil, a woman whose married life was very unhappy, made no progress in her studies, being in the sulks and resentful—as she thought—having been offended.   He decided to make his attitude clear to her, and used his knowledge, acquired in *his* psychoanalysis, about transference and its dangers, for this educational purpose.   He explained to her that too great an intimacy would not aid her studies, but rather hinder them ; as the realisation of the impossibility of marriage would lead to disappointment for both of them.   But in order to show, however, some personal interest in his pupil, he told her certain unimportant details from his own analysis.   Afterwards, however, he thought that he had said perhaps more than he should, more than he wanted to say for the purpose aimed at ;   he himself became apparently subject to the " counter-transference ".   He spontaneously interpreted the following dream, as a *reaction product*, to this affect :

43.   I am sitting opposite a lady from overseas ; at first I am very impersonal, but then after she has made a scientifically correct remark, I am surprised at her knowledge and come closer to her, as if in love.   My wife walks about the room, which naturally embarrasses me.   Then I see Anne as a schoolgirl ;   she is standing in the street and asks whether I would fetch her overcoat quickly from the school building nearby.   I do so, but I am rather upset over her lack of respect for my age.   Then I see my dear Daisy as if it had been *she* who asked me to bring the coat.   I am relieved, but I see with consternation that in addition to her own coat she has another strange coat on.

---

[1] *Int. of Dreams*, Ch. VI.

It is obvious that the manifest dream contains nothing which points quite *openly* to the actual event of the day before. On the other hand it would be, of course, impossible to overlook the existing bearing upon it. In the dream, just as in real life, the dreamer fears that he has gone beyond the necessary reserve, and he regrets having done so in the case of someone in whom he has, in fact, *no* personal interest. The appearance of the beloved Daisy succeeds in calming him ; but this figure, or rather her coat, is changed. It is as if the dream-ego doubted the reality of the consoling substitution ; as if the idea were lurking behind the self-pacification : I am wrong, and I have committed a mistake which can hardly be amended. . . .

It is natural that all the alternating dream figures had their own particular significance for the dreamer. Miss Anne is a charming young girl, who once aroused in him sexual desires which he suppressed quickly for good reasons. Subsequent events proved how right he had been, and how unfortunate it would have been to show even a slight interest in her. The figure Daisy originated from a recent love-affair, in which the dreamer played only a painful, passive rôle, in that his affection was reciprocated insufficiently. He believes that this girl has a bipolar attitude towards him, and that she would soon be able to adjust herself to a new friendship, provided there was a fair chance of an early marriage. The figure of the wife in the dream corresponds with reality. She is the divorced wife of the dreamer, towards whom he has financial obligations, and who thus exerts a continuous inhibiting influence on him. The leading figure in the dream, however, is quite strange to him, as regards both face and appearance ; i.e., we are dealing here with a *new formation* of the dream-work, representing in all probability *all those people and situations* towards whom the dreamer had been obliged to exercise caution throughout his life.

The case shows, like the preceding one, how the actual situation which stimulates the dream, carries out a new distribution of rôles. This example, and its interpretation, shows that for the subconscious often the subjective individual situation matters more than do the particular circumstances and persons, which caused the respective situation of the dreamer on the preceding day. The basic motive of the dream is " caution " in general, not only " caution towards this particular pupil ". Thus, the dream chooses for its effectuated scenery figures *who mean more to him subjectively*, whom he considers more attractive, lovable or more important for himself. At the same time this example shows a symbolic representation of the deplored bipolarity of Daisy. She has *two* coats on (turncoat ?) ; on the one hand, she is perceived as he wants her to be, on the other she carries certain strange surprising traits, she was—if we may turn the old phrase—a sheep in wolf's clothing.

All these examples of dreams confirm at the same time what we said above (Ch. II, (26)) namely, that the basic action, the essence of the real event, represented, or of the endo-psychic process in question, remains more easily recognisable than those parts of the dream which represent " objects " or " persons ". In these instances the person who gave rise to the dream is *completely replaced by others* ; the special way in which the influence of that person occupied the dreamer's mind, appears, however, easily recognisable in the dream.

We have treated of the dream-material from the point of view of the *immediate causation*. We are aware, of course, that the material which has undergone transformation by the dream-work, points to themes which are, at times, far more significant for the individual, than are the recent events which acted as the obvious and immediate dream-stimulus. But the chosen examples were of such a kind, that the actual event in question was itself of a quite important nature, serious enough for the individual, to be treated by the subconsciousness and by the dream-mechanism. *And in relation to these actual events, the pictorial, substituteforming character of the dream was obvious. From this observation we are justified in generalising quite logically on the intensity and extensity of the symbolising process in dreams, and in concluding that intrapsychic processes of other kinds, i.e., complexes and functional contents, will be subject to the same degree of transformation.*

The group of reaction-dreams just treated, are, in their far-reaching tendency towards disguise and substitution, eminently suitable to illustrate the conditions existing in dream symbolism *per se*, and to demonstrate this process in its state of coming into being. They are best fitted to show how far a normal process of transformation can go when the intrapsychic circumstances require. The same conditions with regard to organ-sensation dreams are illustrated by a few examples in Ch. XII, page 218.

CHAPTER IV

FREE ASSOCIATIONS

(1) WHEN free associations are being produced to the various individual elements of the dream, a greater or smaller amount of material is obtained, which relates to the mental life of the dreamer ; it reveals also, to a certain extent, the sources of the dream-image, and at times it may even complete sections of the dream. When the sequence of associations runs smoothly, the bearing of these associations upon the dream, and its various parts, appears fairly obvious ; one gains the impression that these ideas in their abundance are related to the manifest dream as the full text of a book is to the much shorter table of contents.[1] These headings convey similarly only rarely and to an insufficient degree, an idea about the full contents of the respective chapters. Following Freud, the associations are regarded as the " latent dream-thoughts ". This expression implies also the interpretation of this material. The factuality of this mutual relation is beyond all doubt. *But the degree and the particular kind of this relation* is worthy of a closer study ; at any rate, of a more thorough investigation than is presented here ; unfortunately no previous systematic work has been done in this field. When the associations lead to the dream element, either directly or in a more roundabout way, and when it is possible to identify the association with a certain individual dream-element, we might consider any further questions superfluous ; but even then, it might be still problematical whether such an element has been simply fitted into the structure of the dream-image, yet retaining its original content and meaning in the new surroundings ; or whether there is now a *new content associated with the original form.* We shall discuss this question in connection with the following dream :

44. B., a lecturer, while laughing, leans against a chair. We are talking about some accident, referring to a woman.

Associations : B. is generally intelligent, yet not particularly deep or original in thoughts ; but with practical experience.

[1] Cf. Ch. III (32).

He seems to suffer from apparent inferiority feelings, as if realising he is not quite fit for his position, and he often smiles in embarrassment. The " accident " reminds the dreamer of aeroplanes and of travelling overseas. The woman reminds him of a lady who does some acting, quite competently, with an amateur [1] company. He adds : " I do not like pretending to be an important personality ; unfortunately one often has to, because the world demands it. . . ."

The dreamer, who is undergoing training analysis, interpreted the dream, as expressing his own compensated inferiority, as an expression of *his* tendency to pretend to be *somebody*. The day before, someone had said to him that he would undertake a flight overseas without any fear. " I thought," said the dreamer, " that he was only bluffing."

Let us deal with the element referring to the laughing lecturer. When we follow the associations, and accept the interpretation of the dreamer, we find a certain *displacement* has taken place in the significance of the smile. In the dream, it is an ordinary, good-natured laugh ; in the respective association, it is an embarrassed smile. But the dreamer and interpreter explains the smile as that of a man *who wants to appear at ease and good-natured*, in order to stress his importance and self-confidence in the eyes of others. The overt form of the laugh would then be that of a man who *is* apparently at ease, and not of a man who is obviously embarrassed ; though the actual background of his artificial laugh has something to do with embarrassment, i.e., it is meant to cover, or rather to prevent, embarrassment. *In the dream, then, this particular association-element has received, in a certain sense, though not very considerably, a new content.* (Cf. Ch. I, dream 10.)

(2) But what about recollections, thoughts and contents which show only a remote similarity to any part of the manifest dream ? What about associations which, unless they are " interpreted ", show no relation at all to the manifest dream ? Every analyst knows well enough that the sequence of associations sometimes reaches obviously a dream-element only after a long roundabout route, after recollecting a series of elements, which bear no apparent relation to the dream ; until suddenly a thought or a memory comes up whose relation to the original element in the manifest dream appears obvious and self-evident. In such a case the chain of intermediate associations

---

[1] " *Amateur* " *hints at the feeling of* " *insufficiency* ".

seems to be simply a means of approach ; like stations which take us closer to the goal, in time and space, but whose nature doesn't allow us to surmise what this final goal is like. Yet such a conception would seem to call into question the close relation of these " approach associations " to the dream proper. No other satisfactory explanation is possible, therefore, but that every such link in the chain represents only an *external sign* of the *endopsychic approach* towards the genuine dream-element. The position is comparable to that of someone who attempts to listen to events which are occurring behind closed doors ; he hears steps, sounds, movements, indicating that something is happening there ; yet he will hardly be able to guess the complete nature of the various single acts ; though he might have some idea of the goal towards which all these events are tending. Similarly during the act of association, the " retro-grade " process of making conscious the latent dream-thoughts goes on endopsychically in stages ; but not all these " between-stages " are " capable of being thought " or put into word-expression. All the associations are only substitute-ideas for the momentary endopsychic state of the process of " de-composition ". (In such an act of dream-interpretation by means of associations, we proceed in minia-ture, as we do in the gradual analytical " de-composition " and reduction of the whole structure of a neurosis.)

(3) As can be seen here, there exist obvious relations to the law of symbolic substitution in the dream, which has been developed in the previous chapter. The less capable the subconscious complex in question is of " being thought " or of " becoming conscious " at that given moment, the less recog-nisable and the more symbolically disguised must be the conscious substituting element. *In this respect, the chain of associations obviously resembles the process of dream-representation.* Every association-element, then, in its subconscious root, or rather in the " affective nucleus " of this subconscious part (compare in Ch. II) is almost identical with, or at least closely related to, the subconscious affect nucleus of the looked-for dream element. The corresponding conceptual form of the individual association, however, *does not* show this closeness of relation ; it is rather like a word chosen by a person at a loss, when he is unable to find the apt expression, though he is quite aware of *what* he thinks ; (as when somebody says : " You know, it was like a green tree, but it was not quite green, and

it wasn't a real tree, etc."). However, it is small wonder that many associative elements *do* hint, more or less openly, even in their conceptual form, at the genuine content, which latter will only be reached by subsequent associations. That element which approximates in the scs. the character of being " think-able " and of " being conscious ", may be hinted at, even in the conceptual form of the association.

We cite an example, though with considerable omissions ; its extensive discussion would occupy too much space. Every-one who carries out analysis himself, has opportunities for observing *in extenso* the various phenomena prevailing there. Here we want rather to give certain suggestions. This was the dream of a surgeon :

> **45.** Should the content be filled or not ? That was the question in the dream. Perhaps the idea-content of some dream was referred to ?

A typically incomprehensible dream-fragment. The associ-ations run as follows : " I am tired and want to rest. The everyday work of a surgeon demands clear thinking and *it is wonderful not to have to think clearly all the time.* Somehow, this reminds me of a girl I used to know and to like when I was young. She used to roam the fields and woods, and always returned with flowers. *I would have liked to go with her, but did not dare to offer my company.* My memories of this time are beautiful, but I would not like to return to this life-period. Actually, I prefer my present life with all its cares, because *it is filled with real knowledge and real experience.* I think with distaste of my past marriage. . . . I am divorced ; it is not always pleasant to live alone ; but for a certain time such *emptiness* is quite good, a kind of recreation. I sometimes *think of return-ing to my wife* ; but when recollecting *details of the past* I refuse this. Shall I dare marry again ? I feel quite happy alone ; but at the same time full of longing for love and companion-ship. My second wife might want to have children ; should I *fill this second life again with its obligations* ? Yet, cares for children, in fact, constitute the *content of one's life* ; perhaps I should dare to take the step. . . ."

The attentive reader will have noticed the gradual pro-gress, the final clarification in the content of the associations. The relevant phrases are put in italics. As the end of the association-chain shows, we are dealing here with quite a concrete problem which the dreamer has endeavoured, however, to repress from the field of his conscious consideration. In his " free associations ", too, he appears to oscillate between two poles : i.e., either to think the problem through, in all its consequences ; or preferably to enjoy the pleasure of intentional disregard of his problem. This latter tendency is indicated by the phrases : It is wonderful *not to have to think* clearly all the time ; I did *not dare* to offer my company ; for a certain time such *emptiness* is quite good. The other tendency, which strives for an open, clear facing of the problem, is expressed in these phrases : *I would have liked to go with her ; real knowledge and real experience ; to recall details of the past ; to fill* with obligations. At the same time the practical anthitheses are expressed : To marry, and perhaps have children, or not.

The practising analyst, however, will grasp what I mean, and will, during his work, gain deeper insight into that endopsychic process in which the gradual shaping of a consciously thinkable element and the gradual approaching of the respective dream-fragment occur.

(4) *Theoretically* we may postulate, therefore, with certainty the *intrinsic relation of every association to the dream.* But as in the case of the manifest dream, we are here also dealing essentially with the "verbalisation" of a deep psychic process, and must not expect complete congruence ; the various association-elements will approach more or less closely the meaning which is being sought.[1]

It would seem to follow from this that we are justified in *subjecting the associations, too, to the usual symbolic interpretations, as employed with regard to the manifest dream.* We have emphasised repeatedly, and tried to support our assumption, that the transformed subconscious element is expressed in the dream in pictorial fashion ; i.e., everything that is not quite congruent in content and form with the corresponding conscious counterpart is, when entering the dream, represented pictorially. We find a similar condition in the case of associations. There is, too, *an incongruence between the various links of the association-chain and the corresponding endopsychic events.* Essentially the chain of associations represents the imperfect, but gradually successful approach of the dream-element, one is looking for. *Thus every link of this chain carries the character of a substituting symbol.* Theoretically taken, each link of the association-chain repre-

[1] Cf. Ch. I., p. 26.

sents a differently formed substitute of that genuine thought or recollection, which is being looked for as part of the dream-content.   The chain of associations stands in the same relation to the corresponding intrapsychic happening during the act of free association, and at the same time, to the subconscious roots of the dream, as does the pictorially transformed manifest dream to *that* particular subconscious content, which has given rise to the dream, and which former is represented by that dream.

Summarising what has been said so far : The dream-image, as explained, depicts the elements of the *scs.*, in so far as .they differ in content and form from their correlative conscious counterpart, more or less transformed and symbolically disguised.   Yet the associations in their turn are to the investigated dream element, as the various phases of embryonic development are to the mature new-born infant.   In saying this, we have in mind essentially the subconscious, deep endopsychic part of the associative elements ; it is, in fact, this subconscious part of the associative links, which is related to the investigated dream-element through a not quite congruent similarity.   *Thus, here also, the conscious image of these intrapsychic events during the act of association, i.e., the conscious and verbalised association, will constitute only a non-genuine, pictorial representation.*

Every individual link of the subconscious layer of the association-chain is essentially a changed form of the original dream-element, which is being looked for ; *it is an intermediate link which, however, cannot be put into words, and which for that reason is not covered quite congruently by the association as it is verbally expressed by the analysed person.*   This, so I think, finds a certain support from another side.   What we call " *screen-memory*," is fundamentally something quite similar.   A scene is being remembered suddenly, or is retained in consciousness throughout life, as a *substitute-image* of a memory, which itself is repressed because of its painful character for consciousness.[1]

(5) To my knowledge no one as yet has drawn the practical conclusion of trying to treat the associations *systematically* in the same way as is done with the dream proper, i.e., to inter-

---

[1] For instance : A man repeats always automatically " *two and three* ", when he is not occupied with other things.   He considers this just as a kind of childish habit.   He was born in 1902, and he admitted when asked, that he was always curious to know why a *third* child had not come after him ; it was probable that his " song " represented a screen for the problem mentioned.   (The third child could have been born in 1903 . . .)

pret them. I described this procedure first in 1931 (*Psycho-analytische Praxis*, vol. 2) ; and had the satisfaction to see later that Stekel, in his book *Advances of Dream-Interpretation* (1935), mentioned, though only briefly, a similar observation. But he did not deal at length with the problem, nor did he seek to show its background. I will, therefore, repeat in part the arguments which I then advanced ; they were brought forward from a slightly different point of view, which I think is also correct. " As the deep dream is an affective-dynamic process, to which the conceptual level is added as a kind of afterthought, we may assume that the text of the manifest dream constitutes essentially the *first association* to a deeper, ' non-conceptual ' content. Manifest dream-image and chain of associations, therefore, are on the same level in relation to the deep, non-conceptual dream-processes. . . .[1] On examining several *dream-series* I found that the associations permit of the same kind of symbolic interpretation as is practised analytic-ally in the case of the dream proper. In this manner we gain new insight, and also more essential confirmation of our interpretation of the manifest dream."

(6) The following fragment occurred in the dream of a man who was suffering from an obsessional feeling of lack of independence :

46. I am looking for something, when I see my friend X repairing the leg of an easy-chair. I think he is doing this for me. . . .

Associations : " Yesterday I accompanied my father on a visit to a friendly family ; he left his walking-stick there. It remained hanging from an easy-chair. . . . The chair was defective, and I wondered why it was left in that state. I myself never mend anything that is broken in our household ; all that is done, or ordered to be done, by my aunt. . . ."

According to this last association, the aunt should be substituted for the friend X. Indeed, this aunt constitutes the patient's most important support in life. His clumsiness was arranged, or at least exaggerated, in order to justify and make more secure his close relation to this self-sacrificing aunt. *The leg of the chair signifies a " firm foothold " ; in its defective state it*

---

[1] Frequently a forgotten part of the dream, or even some older dream, will appear during the process of association. This, too, shows the fundamental identity of dream and free association. Cf. dreams 2 and 3. *Cf. also p. 141.*

is a symbol of lack of manly independence. The father's walking-stick can be interpreted similarly as the principle of firmness and directness, as the " rod of correction and exhortation " (in the language of the Bible).[1] After this symbolic interpretation of the associations, we find that the original cause of the close relation with the aunt becomes much clearer. It was the disturbed father-son relationship (" the stick has got *lost* ; it is hanging from the *defective* easy-chair "). The father had married a second time, and had little affection left for his children ; the aunt in question had been treated by the father with a similar lack of consideration and affection. We do not propose to go into the remainder of the determining conditions of the dream ; our purpose was only to show the possibility and fruitfulness of a symbolic interpretation of the associations.

An obsessional patient, who was treated with full success, suffered from the very painful obsession that *if* he should once marry, this marriage would cause his death. This dream occurred near the beginning of the treatment :

> **47.** I saw my late brother, very well dressed. He had on a very distinctive hat. Then a drunkard tried to beat me.

Associations : " My brother was really very pedantic. Once someone made a critical remark about his hat ; he immediately bought a new one. My father once bought a hat for himself, and at the same time one for my brother. *The hat my father bought for himself then, looked like the one my brother wore in the dream.* Once I bought myself a hat instead of the cap which I used to wear. I did not have permission to buy it, and my mother threatened to smack me. Once I went home with my late brother and my mother, and a drunken man threatened to beat us." The analysis revealed the following main causes of the patient's suffering :

(i) Hatred against the father, who terrorised the family. (He identifies him with the dead brother ; " the hat in the dream was like that of the father ".)

(ii) A strong feeling of guilt towards the mother. Once he wanted to marry a girl against her will ; she said threateningly : " This must not happen as long as I live." Thus, the planned marriage became associated with the death of his mother.

---

[1] *Proverbs*, Chs. XXII and XXIX.

The association referring to the mother who threatens and beats him, can *also* be understood symbolically : I am beaten, cursed by my mother. She prevents my buying a new hat = reaching my libidinous aim (hat = male genitals and rôle of husband).

The association regarding the hats, bought at the same time for father and brother, signify symbolically : *Just as my brother has no hat any longer* (*i.e., no genitals and no life*) *so should my father be without one.* (In fact, the patient admitted such thoughts quite consciously.)

The sentence in his associations which deals with the threat of the drunkard to his brother, to his mother and to himself, signifies symbolically : " My mother and I might die in a similar manner to my brother." (He had once had homosexual relations with his brother, and thought he had injured him in some way. In his opinion, he perhaps killed the brother through his sexuality, and might do the same to his mother, if he married. Then he would have to die too, for punishment.) *All the complexes which I discovered through interpretation of the associations were also confirmed in other ways, and admitted by the patient.*

The following dream was reported by a patient who suffered from anxiety, and who felt some indigestion at the time of the dream :

> **48.** A lady friend of mine sends me butter by an ugly servant. A letter is also included. I don't believe that she has really written this charming letter. . . .

Associations : " My stepmother used to like eating pastries made with butter. Yet, as they caused her stomach pains she used to prepare them only for us children."

This association makes it likely that the neurotic sickness of the patient (indicated by " stomach pains ") is somehow related to the person of the stepmother. Earlier dreams had made me suspect a pathological positive fixation to this stepmother. The patient denied this. The association given above, makes it quite clear, if symbolically transformed : " The stepmother gives me her love (pastries)."

(7) The fact that associations carry a symbolic content seems thus assured. But that does not mean necessarily that in any given case the symbolic meaning will give more information and understanding of the dream and of the whole situation,

than the literal meaning of the association. Theoretically, we might assume : the further the literal meaning is from the dream-element proper, the more useful should the symbolic interpretation prove. The examples quoted, however, do *not* support this assumption ; rather on the contrary. I believe that at the present state of our knowledge we cannot make any final statement. Just as there are various and diverse types of dreamer, a fact which is somehow connected with character-type and psychic constitution, so it is certain that the kind and relation of associations to the manifest dream also varies.[1] Just as there are people who dream a great deal (we analysts do not welcome this during treatment), so there are people who associate more or less freely. Some types associate " close to the dream-element ", others at some distance from it. Some associations are related to some subordinate layer of the dream element ; not to that which is of central interest for the illness. Limitation of the field of associations by occasional active interference, as Stekel, Jung and Bjerre suggest, seems to be indispensable, if one does not propose to extend the treatment indefinitely.

We must take into account that theoretically the dream contains hereditary, infantile, present and prospective aspects. Also, included is the attitude to the analyst, which depends largely on the genuine " reproductive transference of previous constellations ", although it also must have, in every case, an individual, additional note. After all, the therapist is different from his " predecessors " in the mental past of the patient. Thus every dream-element contains the *affect-value of all these aspects*. And for the same reason, the associations will refer now to this content, now to that content, of the dream. Hence the well-known experience that abundant associations can become a very apt means of " evasion ". (See Ch. IX, on the analytical situation as reflected in the free associations.)

(8) The stimulating rôle of a leading motif, or a guiding aim in the production of free associations, is borne out by the following observation. If there are two or more dreams remembered from the same night, and one succeeds in gaining a longer series of associations to each of them, in some cases there appear obviously similar elements in the individual association-groups. More exactly : there is either a motif common to the different manifest dreams ; or a motif common

---

[1] Cf. pp. 21–2, p. 143, p. 146, p. 231 and p. 240.

to one manifest dream and to the association-chain pertaining to another dream ; or finally, there is an obviously common motif in each group of associations, arrived at from the different dreams of the same night. The following example will illustrate the last mentioned possibility :

(*a*) A *woman* comes from a door holding in her arm a *thin baby* . . .

(*b*) A friend of mine is stooping over some square thing, and tries to lift it, it is very heavy . . .

Associations to the first dream-fragment : Mrs. S. is a very gay woman ; she is friendly and *helpful*, but strongly *polygamous*. The baby reminds the dreamer of a visit as a schoolboy to a museum, where he was shown the picture of a historical personality of medieval times, who was imprisoned for life for *unfaithfulness*. There was also a skeleton of an *infant*, and the young student had the impression that it was the remainder of an *illegitimate child* of that lady. . . .

Associations to the second dream : The friend suffers from slight depressions. He is very *helpful* towards the dreamer. He seems to like his young wife, yet at the same time *he glances at any young girl* who passes. . . . The friend reminds the dreamer of his father, who was also very *much impressed by smart and high-standing women.* The dreamer thought in his childhood, that *he was not the child of his parents*, but that he was adopted by them. His mother was strictly moral and conservative but always tired and excited. She did very much for her children, but at the same time, she was unhappy in her marriage. She was " mentally never married " but remained the child of her parents. . . .

The motif of the " polygamous woman " and the " sideglancing friend " are obviously similar. But not less similarity exists between the motif of the " illegitimate child " in the first sequence, and " the mother who mentally refuses to put up with having a husband and children " in the other. The fantasy of being only adopted, runs along the same line. . . .

True, such obvious similarities are to be found only in the associations of individuals, who produce them freely and abundantly, and more or less " near to the element " looked for. However, at times the symbolic interpretation of some association reveals the presence of such common elements. The similarity appears obvious, after one certain association has been replaced by its symbolic substitute.

A few more interesting instances have been described in " The different dreams of the same night ". The common motifs point to some central problems of the individual under analysis. We propose to deal with this aspect in detail in our " Special Dream-Interpretation ".

CHAPTER V

THE WORLD OF DREAMING AND OF DREAMS

(1) WE now enter a field which, at first, seems capable of illumination only by the unreal light of hypothesis and phantasy. The investigations which could be carried out in the fields explored hitherto, relate to the dream-image, to the remembered part of the dream, to elements which after awaking have become part of conscious thought through memory, and which thus have become open to subjective introspection of the dreamer, and capable of objective analysis. But we are naturally *not* in a position to observe our dreams introspectively, and to investigate them analytically, while we are asleep and actually still dreaming. We are not in a position, cognitively, to grasp the *act of dreaming*, and the dream-image itself, *in statu nascendi*. True, we *do* experience the dream, and during less profound sleep, also in a way, the dreaming-process, the birth-pangs of the dream. But the dream-ego—or the dream-con-sciousness, as Sante de Sanctis called it—is *not* accessible to investigation in a direct manner. It is only the dream-image which is accessible, i.e., the sum of the dream-contents, and the total " strange world " which has been created and shaped from these dream-elements, and into which the latter appear to have been set. What we *can* state about this world is but to note its similarity to, and its deviations from, the world of waking life.[1] The individual elements of the dream correspond in principle and phenomenologically with those of waking life. Yet, the *quality of experiencing* far outweighs that of thinking and of reflection. I think, also, that *the separated position of the experiencing ego* is not so clearly marked within the dream as in waking life. I have already pointed out that this is a conse-quence, of the fact that the whole dream represents actually various parts of the ego itself. I have also noted that the difference between the two kinds of experiencing can be grasped subjectively ; we seem to undergo a *true experience* while dreaming ; but the quality of this experiencing, as compared to that in waking life, is definitely less distinct. What, however, constitutes the vividness or rather the experi-

[1] Cf. Ch. II (17).

enced *intensity* of our dreaming, is the preponderance of the *emotional factor*, as indeed every investigator has emphasised. *One* cause for the difference in quality which distinguishes the two kinds of experiencing, then, appears to be the preponderance of the cognitive, of the clearly formulated thought-element in the case of waking experiencing, and that of the rather vague, affective element in the case of dreaming. The other cause lies in the fact that, as mentioned above, both the dreaming ego and its whole surroundings are only representations of events within the dreamer's psyche ; i.e., that *ego and its surroundings in the dream are one.*

(2) The *affective element in dreaming* deserves a special and more detailed treatment. First of all, let us bear in mind the conception propounded in previous chapters, that the " deep " dream-process proper is a non-conceptual, and only affect-energetic event, because the " molecular elements " of the psychic disposition are connected comparatively loosely with their conceptual counterparts, and thus, the " conceptualisation " and " verbalisation " of the dream is a separate process. This hypothesis readily explains the fact which has just been stressed, viz., that the dream is " felt " rather than " thought ". There is, however, something more to it than this. One's own ego is being perceived in waking life too, rather by *feeling it* than by *thinking of it.* But as the whole dream deals with the ego, i.e., it has the conditions of the ego as its essential subject, it is only natural that in dreaming, too, the affective element of experiencing prevails.

This latter consideration, and the previously mentioned conception of the affect-energetic nature of dreaming, are complementary, and constitute *one* single factor. The present author looks upon this formulation, and its support by arguments and proofs, as the fundamental thesis of the dream-theory, especially for the psychotherapist. In the course of our expositions and explanations, we have referred to this thesis whenever necessary and fruitful. In general, so I believe, it might give the young medical man a deeper understanding of the " *concrete* " *nature* of psychic processes, and thus, of the marked influence of mental processes on the somatic aspect of the organism.

(3) Here we propose to deal first of all with the analytical process in its intra-psychic aspect, and in so far as it expresses itself in dreams. Since the essence of the analytical situation,

and of the analytical process, is to be found in the field of the individual's affective life, and the de-composing influence of this method is essentially concerned with the individual's emotional world, it is only natural to suppose that the same influence of the analysis exerts its special effect also on the formation of dreams. Elements of the subconscious and of the dream-ego react more readily to the analytical process than do those of consciousness, because in consequence of the looser connection with the conceptual component, their affective counterpart is more *in statu nascendi.*[1] They are becoming mobilised and driven farther in the direction of formativeness, i.e., they are made "capable of being thought" and of "becoming conscious". Hence, as explained elsewhere, the increased production of dreams in the course of analysis. (Ch. I (8).)

We can also explain on these grounds the nature of the so-called transference-dreams. It is by experience established that *the dream always indicates the analytic situation,* apart from the historical significance of the elements, and apart from the functional significance they carry with regard to the mental life of the dreamer. According to whether the inner attitude of the patient towards the analyst, and towards his efforts, is positive or negative, and according to the special quality of the affective attitude displayed towards him at any particular stage of the treatment, the verbalised dream also will contain a corresponding allusion. Here, for instance, is a dream which demonstrates this quite clearly :

49. I am having an interesting conversation with my friend . . .

And again, in another case :

50. There was a lively discussion in the hospital, which I enjoyed very much . . .

Or in a third case :

51. I meet my dear friend, and full of joy we shake hands . . .

However historical the individual dream-elements may be, however close and obvious their bearing upon the other (non-analytical) spheres of the individual's life, such a dream-image represents *at the same time* implicitly a symbol of the

---

[1] This means here, as in chemistry, a state of "newness" with increased reactivity.

analytical attitude obtaining at that moment. (Cf. Ch. IX.) This is so, not only because as we know the dream is full of condensations, i.e., over-determined in its sources, but also because the depth-process during treatment, i.e., the analytical affective condition, gains easy access to the affect-energetic layer of the dream-process ; and thus, it decidedly participates in determining the formation of dreams ; furthermore, because the conceptual content of the dream represents only " verbalisations " of the affective elements mentioned and of their combinations respectively (we describe the assumed facts only schematically). Thus, the transference-situation gains influence more quickly and intensely on the *scs.* and on the dream, than on the sphere of conscious thinking and feeling ; not only because a certain resistance and a certain repression fight against the conscious " transference " ; but also because, as pointed out, the very conditions of the " affect-energetic dreaming " are more favourable, and more susceptible for being influenced by the transference-affect. I do not forget, of course, that the transference-affects and their variations arise from the subconscious and its complexes, i.e., that the " transference-dream " is only a secondary, mirroring product ; what I had here in mind was the *primary* exogenous influence of the analyst as a " human being " exerted on the person analysed. This influence is not too dependent on certain individually coloured complexes and attitudes ; this impression comes into operation independently of the pre-existent subconscious attitudes, and finds, as mentioned above, easier access to the affect-energetic dreaming-process than to the conscious thought and conscious feelings of the person analysed. Hence, even the slightest transference becomes fairly obvious in the dream. We have identified in all these considerations, the " subconsciousness " with " dream-consciousness " and " dream-ego " ; schematically, this is justified for the purposes of our exposition ; although I am quite aware that the *dream-conscious* constitutes only a part of the whole *scs. system.*

(4) Earlier authors have regarded the affectivity as the central problem of the dream. De Sanctis said quite rightly : " The motor of the dream is the affective state ; its driving force is the expression of affective energy. . . . The affective state in the dream is a *free* one ; through sleep, it becomes independent of the fetters and claims of reality. . . . One should, however, not forget that this is only a general view-

point. In every particular case one finds incidental features which take their origin from associations, from the interference of actual feelings, and from partial influences of thought and logic as far as these can be reconciled with the oscillations in the depth of sleep " (Chapter on the " Dynamism of the Dream "). Stekel also remarked in his *Language of Dreams* : " The dream is not a play of thought, but a struggle of affects."

The conception suggested here, however, has in view the *formed affective components of the ideas*, and consequently, for us, the dream-content in its manifest form too, is something determined and " intended ", not something merely accidental, as it was for de Sanctis, who also said : " The affective state is capable of forming the same material either into a dream-tragedy or into a dream-comedy." On the basis of analytic experience it is impossible to believe in such a lack of determination, and scientific thinking refuses to subscribe to it. It is true that the depth of sleep, for instance, or the endopsychic state, or " organic " factors (though influencing the psyche, see below) *may* influence the dream-image ; but in that case the image *is* in fact determined, and there is no longer " the same material ".

We may recollect here once more (though for some readers such repetitions might be tiresome) that any mental element which has undergone in the *scs.* an essential change—i.e., even in its " affect-energetic nucleus ", appears in the dream-image symbolically represented or replaced by an associative image. Also, the multiform changes of symbols in the dream-series which relate to the *same* complex, correspond certainly with changes and variations in content, of the " affect-energetic nucleus " of the respective idea in the *scs.*

The following remark by Havelock Ellis seems to me very suggestive in this connection : " Sleep is especially favourable to the *production of emotion*, because while it allows a considerable amount of activity to sensory processes, and a very wide freedom to the imagery founded on sensory activities, it largely and in many directions *inhibits motor activity*. The action suggested by sensory exitation cannot, therefore, be carried out. As soon as the impulse enters motor channels it is impeded, broken up, and scattered in a vain struggle. *This process is transmitted to the brain as a wave of emotion . . ."* This may sound like a pretty theory. But the extensive inhibition of motor activity during sleep is a fact ; and so is the heightened affectivity of the dream, on the other hand. Perhaps their interdependence should not be rejected entirely. I shall try in the following section to develop a similar idea ; yet it deals with the *more extensive problem of the sources of the dream*, and it will, I think, prove helpful for gaining a unitary point of view which may be universally acceptable.

(5) The dream is a psycho-affective event ; Freud has shown this to be true beyond the possibility of doubt. The older theories, which had seen in the dream merely the expression of vegetative stimulation, coupled with " dissociated thought-elements ", had to give way. The organic stimulus was recognised as an *additional factor* in the dream-formation, and the motive power of this dream-formation was reduced on the one hand to the libido (Freud), on the other to the affect as such (de Sanctis, Havelock Ellis), to the élan vital (Bergson), or to the total psycho-affective world of subconscious spheres (Stekel).

Yet we can hardly pass over so lightly the wealth of vegetative stimuli in their rôle as a source of the dream. When we then ask for the exact position of the *affect*, we are again led in the same direction. James [1] had stated long ago that we can cognise the affective state only in its bodily localisation. " Bodily changes follow directly the perception of the exciting act, and . . . our feeling of the same changes as they occur, *is the emotion*." [2] As I once said schematically, *the affect lies at the meeting point of " soma " and " psyche "*. It is called forth by psychic stimuli, and it is a psychic experience ; but one that takes place in the organic sphere, and the energy of which, in all probability, originates there. Its " energy " comes into being as a result of a particular peripheral organic stimulation, and its diverse subjective nuances are a consequence of the multiform combinations of multilocular excitation in the various somatic regions (muscles and skin included).

---

[1] *The Principles of Psychology*, 1905.

[2] His original theory, as is well known, stated that the external perception of a certain situation brings about first the bodily changes, and only the experience of these sensations creates secondarily the mental emotion. This concept had to undergo a considerable change, for different reasons. Sherrington and others could show that, at least in the animal, the interruption of the sympathetic pathways leading to and from the internal organs, does not render emotional behaviour impossible. But, as I intend to show in a special work, the *elaborated emotional feeling*, though accompanied by a distinct " psychic " counterpart, and though primarily originating in thalamic regions, always contains this vegetative-organogenic component, provided that the unity of bodily organisation is preserved. (Cf. Ch. X.)

Superficial investigation suffices to recognise a whole series of affect-localisations ; heart, abdomen, mucous membrane of the mouth, and skin—all these come into the foreground of subjective perception in cases of psychic excitement. But why should we forget all those somatic regions whose stimulation cannot be observed by direct introspection ? It is hardly possible to assume that psychic stimulation extends *only* to the regions mentioned ; it seems much more likely in principle that the whole organism, with all its individual systems, can be thrown into excitement by the psychic stimulus, and *give rise to affective energy in its turn.* The important contribution of physically stimulated organic regions, both to the dream-material and to the emotional element in the dream, suggests that the normal, not increased, organ stimuli, play an important part in the dream-formation and *in the production of the physiological affective states* of the personality. For the psycho-analyst the existence of the so-called organ-libido, the psychic cathexis of the organs, is a self-evident fact. But to my mind it seems to be just as well established that *every living, " affective " mental content is reflexively related in the organisation of the personality with certain organic regions and certain organic functions.* In other words, fear does not simply " influence " the heart and the blood-circulation as an externally noxious stimulus ; the complex " fear " *belongs*, intrinsically and permanently to the system of circulation ; and stimulation of the " fear-complex " constitutes at the same time automatically an excitement for a certain kind of circulatory reaction.[1] And it is not only the heart, or the alimentary canal, the skin, or the musculature which possess their psycho-affective correlates, but *all the organic regions, and also, separately, all the various organic functions of the same region.* A traumatic disturbance of such a psychic element implies automatically a certain disturbance, even if subliminal, of a corresponding organic function. *The affect-energy originates in the organ, in the periphery, because these regions possess a psychic component, because their essence contains also a certain psycho-affective quality. Organic stimuli, increased in intensity, influence the dream only because they play in any case a normal part in the origin of dreams ;* because the dream always and in every image is a " representation of organic events ". And this again is so because *organic energy implies at the same time psycho-*

---

[1] This is only a schematic example ; there are many different kinds of " fear ", and the circulatory apparatus itself is also a very complicated unity.

affective content.[1] I am convinced that every dream in its totality originates as much in the organs [2] (viz., in the libidinal organ-cathexis) as in the " purely psychic affective " sources. In reality, one might say that the boundaries become effaced and leave only *one* material for the dream-formation, viz., the affect-energetic one ; only *one* motive source of dreaming : the psycho-affective world of the personality. This world embraces the total personality, both in its mental and physical aspect. But this latter is already a fairly old, almost banal idea. During sleep, when conscious thought disappears and the psyche turns away from reality and sense-perception, this *organic affectivity* seems to grow stronger ; or perhaps the *dream-ego* is more apt to perceive this element. In favour of this hypothesis we might cite the fact that organic disturbances of subliminal intensity are perceived in the dream, long before there is a conscious perception of them. Be that as it may, it is primarily the heightened " affective quality " of the dream which we have sought to make more understandable. This heightening is due to " organ-energy " which splits off affective quality [3] and supplies it to the dream-process. It is easy to see that *organic stimulation and motor-energy have something in common* ; thus the assumption that heightened emotionality in the dream is due to inhibited or transformed motor energy (as suggested by H. Ellis) fits in well with our theory. At the beginning we pointed out that what the dream *experiences*, is the ego itself, and consequently this dream experience is *felt* rather than imagined or thought. Now we have shown *how*, i.e., by which means and ways *this feeling-function* operates.

(6) At this point we intend to discuss a problem which is

[1] G. R. Heyer in a lecture on " The treatment of the psyche through influencing the body " * suggested that there is a constant inherent relation between certain organ-systems and equivalent mental forces. " The gastro-enteral system carries the principle of preserving and protecting the individual, by depriving heterogen food-material of its foreign ' mana ', and imparting to it the specific human rhythm of life. The circulatory system carries the ' self-ego ' and its stability."

The similarity of this philosophical conception to that developed in this work is obvious. Yet it is also clear that the author of this work arrived in his *independent* research at his broader affect-biological conception by study of the dream-world, by enquiring into the close and ramified relationship obtaining between the continuous physiological processes and the richness and the consequent large variety of the dream-world.

[2] Older authorities have, of course, recognised the great importance of organic events for the dream-formation, but they did not see that it was the psycho-affective element of the organs and their functions which matter.

[3] Cf. Ch. X.

* VI. *Kongressbericht für Psychotherapie.* (Report on the sixth Congress for Psychotherapy.)

of great importance to the psychotherapist in his capacity as dream-interpreter ; *the evaluation and interpretation of the emotion in the dream.* In this connection we do *not* refer to the heightened affect-quality of the dreaming-experience as a whole, which was discussed above ; but we mean the individual, " formed " affect-reactions (emotions) within the dream event. One notices sometimes that persons who do not mean much to us in waking life, become highly important in the dream ; their little faults and weaknesses, their small sins of omission and commission which they have perpetrated against us, all these features might be heavily underlined in the dream. (Cf. dream 11 on B's deceitfulness.) Similarly, we may rejoice, or be dejected, because of events which would be much less emotionally experienced in waking life. Analytical experience suggests two possible explanations. One alternative is that the dream is indicative of the attitude of the deeper subconscious towards the point in question ; this attitude, as existing in the subconscious world of thought and feeling, is characterised by greater intensity and extensity. A slight degree of a sentiment, operating in consciousness, as of criticism, fear, or any interest, may mean *far more* for the subconscious, and therefore for the real affective world of the individual, than it signifies to the conscious mind, which is a controlled, limited and directed thinking. We mean, it is diverted from the inner complexes and directed towards logical aspects. One might also say that in such cases, associative links, which, however, remain unconscious, exert their intensifying effect on the dream-level. One has the impression that *the dream continues, widens and strengthens the conscious element.*

The other possibility is, that the persons and actions of such a dream are only screen-images, replacing, in fact, a different complex, which latter is actually of greater importance for the ego ; the original affect, however, is retained even after association with these newly formed screen-elements. " The dreamwork transforms contents more easily than the affects pertaining to the former ; the affects themselves appear sometimes very resistant." (Freud in *Introductory Lectures*, Ch. XIV.) This is one of the most important problems which the therapist encounters in the course of his work. According to Freud and Stekel,[1] it has always proved most fruitful to keep to the special *emotion* accompanying the dream-experience

[1] Freud, *Int. of Dreams*, Ch. VI, and Stekel, *Dic. Spr. des Traumes*, Ch. XIV.

when interpreting the dream.   But I want to emphasise that those cases in which intense anxiety is coupled with an apparently harmless content, are very *rare* in my experience.[1]   (For instance : one dreams with great anxiety that he eats an apple.)   They are much rarer in any case, than the reverse possibility where the expected and reasonable affect does not occur in spite of a suitable content.   (For instance : one dreams about a horrifying event, murder or a putrefying corpse, without experiencing the appropriate emotion.)   The feeling of anxiety is a factor which leads to awakening ;   accordingly, the dream-content which is associated to it, must assume a form which more or less corresponds to such an emotion, in accordance with the working mode of the conscious system. Even though the dream-image may often transform and express symbolically that psychic complex, which is the true source of the dream-anxiety, it is still generally an image, which for conscious thought as well, appears troublesome and makes us feel uneasy.   It may be a dream-situation involving danger— either to the dreamer or displaced to someone else—or a furious quarrel, an examination or some other precarious situation ;   the dream-image suits the quality of the affected reaction, in principle at least.   This behaviour is similar to that of dreams which lead to pollution or orgasm often containing appropriate *openly* erotic scenes.   Once I had a female patient who used to dream, that as she was running along the highway she had orgasm-like sensations.   This rare type of dream corresponds with the fact of reality that adolescents may, at times, experience actually sexual feelings during different states of expectation or tension, *which latter are not of an erotic nature* ;   for instance, in running, in games or during an examination.   But in general, feelings of orgasm accompanying the dream, *are* connected with adequate dream-images ; if my memory serves me right, this is always the case with male pollution-dreams (there is at least a certain person present or hinted at).   Erection-dreams, however, are frequently completely disguised.   As explained above, similar correspondence is true of anxiety dreams ;   and this congruity between affect and content holds of all dreams accompanied by painful emotional reactions.

(7) But there is a need to dwell longer on the phenomenon

---

[1] Dreams of embarrassment because of minor deficiencies in dress are, of course, " justified ", motivated.

of development of anxiety during sleep. When anxiety is aroused by dyspepsia, circulatory disturbances, or by blocking of the respiratory apparatus (mucus in the throat, nose stuffed up, or face covered), the accompanying dream can be readily explained as a simple process of " objectification " and " dramatisation " of the organic events. Naturally, even there, the conceptual dream-content is always capable of analysis and of reduction to its primal sources ; and such a dream can thus be explained in its relation to the psychic ego. *However, the affect which is associated with it seems to be primarily " organ-anxiety ".* And thus, there might arise the doubt whether or not *every* anxiety-dream comes about in a similar manner ; one could feel obliged to assume that anxiety-dreams originate on the basis of minor organic dysfunctions, not recognisable as such. If this be so, we would have to conclude that the emotional reaction, accompanying the dream, carries no reliable significance guiding the analyst in interpreting the dream-content, as claimed by Freud and Stekel. Our " psycho-analytical sentiment ", of course, struggles against such a generalisation ; we know too well that *there are*, undoubtedly, anxiety states conditioned by mental causes ; and, therefore, we might assume them to occur similarly in dreams. Yet, the doubt in every individual dream-case remains, and at first quite justifiedly.

The possible answer, that it is in every case the same physiological mechanism which effectuates the anxiety state, does not promise any information about the primary cause and source of this emotional reaction ; it does not suggest whether in a certain case it is a mental conflict or alternatively an organic disturbance, which is primarily at work. One should, in such cases, always bear in mind incipient coronary diseases, or coronary spasms.

For the psychotherapist in his capacity as dream interpreter, such distinction may be important at times. For, if a dream content, or a complex lying behind such a dream, leads to anxiety, and does it by reason of its own nature, then we can be sure that the respective complex carries a pathogenic power and significance. If, however, a complex *does not* lead to anxiety feelings, or to overt symptoms, then, though its existence is clearly suggested by any dream, it is merely present ; yet its rôle and its influencing value have first to be proved by further analysis of the remaining circumstances.

There is, of course, a middle way. The organic feeling of displeasure draws towards itself an appropriate psychic material, a material which itself originates from conflicts of the individual and is, therefore, capable of producing affect ; such mental content is, in fact, always present. Thus, the psychoanalyst can tackle such dream-material in the same way as he does the usual anxiety-dreams which, according to their content, deal individual psychic complexes. We cannot rest here, however, but must pursue our question further. What is the exact relation of the organic event to the anxiety-feeling, and thus to the dream-content ? Let us give a few examples of this type of dream :

> **52.** A lady dreamed that her husband called her aside and said : " Now don't scream, I am going to tell you something. *I have to kill a man. It is necessary to put him out of his agony !* " He then showed her a young man lying on the floor, with a wound in his breast, and covered with blood. He took something and leaned over the man. She turned aside and heard a horrible gurgling sound. Then all was over. They made the body into a parcel and *with terrible difficulty and effort the wife assisted her husband* to get the body downstairs. . . . She had all along been full of apprehension lest the deed should be discovered, and before waking in terror, she was looking out of the window at a large crowd which surrounded the house with shouts of " Murder " and threats.

" The tragedy was built up out of a few impressions received during the previous day ; none of them contained any suggestion of murder. The tragic element appears to have arisen entirely from a *supper of pheasant.* To account for our oppression during sleep, sleeping consciousness assumes moral causes, which alone appear to it of sufficient gravity to be adequate to the immense emotions we are experiencing." (Havelock Ellis, *The World of Dreams*, ch. on " Emotions in Dreams ".) The same person is reported to have dreamed 10 years later, after another pheasant-dinner, of " murder " again ; this time, however, it was she who was to be killed.

Here is another example :

> **53.** Someone invited me for dinner, but it was all very strange. I had suspicions they wanted to *poison* me. I went to a doctor, but was *afraid* he might keep something from me.

A third, different example :

> **54.** My mouth is full of mucus. Disgusting ! Like raw meat. *I want to be sick.*

And a fourth example, of yet a different type :

> 55. I see my sister, pale and old. Beside her is a fresh, youthful girl, but she is just as old as my sister. Then some-one—a third woman—has something wrong with her ; there is a rectal inspection. But I don't see the person ; only the anus. (Wakes up with dyspepsia.)

(8) The explanation will appear quite easy to the psycho-logist with psychoanalytical orientation and experience. He will be familiar with the cannibalistic, necrophilic, scatalogic and other " disgust-complexes " which, in some rare analyses, play an important part, and which may become conscious and manifest in certain psychopathic individuals. Once I treated a refined colleague for impotency ; he had many scatalogic phantasies, and used to imagine himself as fæces sliding down the bowels of another person. It is, of course, well known that all the ideas of " incorporation ", desire, elimination and dis-gust are closely related to the *idea of the alimentary tract*. As we pointed out above, they are in reality *psychic correlates, psychic contents, " cathexes of the organic system in question."* Similarly, ideas and images related to danger to one's life, are closely associated with the circulatory system, and with other vital centres in the organic structure. Our description here is naturally merely schematic ; but it is hoped that the reader will understand the point referred to.[1]

An organic disturbance, then, implies and signifies in probability the simultaneous stirring up of the associated complexes. Their psychoanalytic investigation and interpretation is, therefore, quite justified ; though their possible origin from, or depend-ence on, organic processes is in principle admitted. For all practical aspects, there is little difference whether, for instance, an " incorporation-complex " (this means the incorporation-phantasy, conscious or subconscious, related to beloved, living objects), or other different kinds of such mental elements, are founded on a constitutional structure, or acquired by individual experiences of the patient, or split off from, and supplied by, a special " organic source ". The difference for practical

---

[1] One of my psychotic patients suffers from the monosymptomatic hypo-chondriac delusion that he does not pass sufficient urine and fæces. He is aware of having a daily motion but he " feels that he is still full ". Such cases, and many similar, show clearly that there exists a separate psychic content of the organs, which appears in the self-perception, to be " detached, loosened " from its material counterpart. There remains in the ego-perception of such indi-viduals a dissatisfaction with regard to the *psychic* counterpart of the whole excretion complex.

analysis lies *only* in the more temporary character of the latter contribution, and in the more ingrained nature of the first mentioned possibility.

In parenthesis, I should like to point out that we can well imagine in principle the causal derivation of various, though more primitive, complexes from the organic spheres ; e.g., that the scatalogic complex could somehow be split off, " excreted " from the cathexis of the intestine (this denotes the psycho-affective content of the latter). I do not know how far other authors have dealt with this possibility. It is obvious that this assumption presents a firm foundation for developing a valid theory of the organ-choice of differently shaped neuroses.

We must imagine, then, that the normally functioning organ splits off " affective-energy ", and that this constitutes the normal contribution of the organ to the dream-formation.[1] The over-stimulated organ, however, produces an overdose of affect, and also more " abnormal complexes " of the kind described above. The liberation of these affect-energetic elements is felt as a strong threat by the sleeping ego exceeding its regulative, assimilative powers. This might explain the intense feeling of " being endangered " in the corresponding dream-contents. The underlying organic process itself is, in fact, almost *never* such which involves a real threat to the dreamer's life. (Coronary disease, which also often causes painful dreams, is an exception to this rule.) During the sleeping state and in dreaming we perceive the *freed* " *complex-energy* ", which in virtue of its *status nascendi* (intense reactive force) constitutes a threat to the assimilative capacity of the psychic mechanism. At that point awakening interrupts the process.

(9) We now continue our discussion of the world of dreams. The placid, natural acceptance of things and events which contradict the world of logical thoughts, is the most striking phenomenon which attracted the attention of all pre-analytic observers. The " absurdity " of the dream has been dealt with thoroughly by Freud, who also made an attempt to explain it. (Cf. his sections on dream-distortion and on absurdity.) The work of the analyst, i.e., the reduction of the manifest dream to the latent dream-thoughts, enables him to transform this nonsense into sense. But this method of explaining the nonsense implies the dismemberment of the manifest dream. *We cannot, however, deny that the manifest dream is an autonomous*

[1] Cf. Ch. X.

structure, and consequently we have to come to terms with the lack of logic of the dream as a whole.[1] The simplest assumption is, that the dream-ego knows the latent dream-thoughts, and so replaces automatically and intra-psychically the dream by the details which lie at the back of it. Thus there is no real need to be " astonished ". (There are, however, rare cases in which the dreamer realises the " absurdity " and " impossibility " of the dream-event ; such cases were explained as " interference " by the waking system of the dreaming.)

The following theory seems to me to approach much more closely the facts. The dream (except where it deals with real relations to the external world) is fundamentally a *representation of the whole ego.* What appears to us as nonsense and lack of logic, is really only the *pictorial expression of endopsychic and somatic events, which, of course, are not subject to the laws of our logic. Therefore, the dreamer has no reason to be astonished or to object to the dream-events.* His dream-ego knows with what it is dealing. This, of course, is *not* the point of view of the interpreting psychoanalyst. He is primarily interested in the relation of the dream-elements to conscious thinking, feeling and experiencing. Consequently, he is forced to look for the associations to the dream-elements, and he is thus often enabled to resolve the apparent contradictions. But the manifest dream in its totality, as a specific product of the subconscious, seems also to have, in virtue of its unity, its *own logical laws.* We succeed but rarely, by a kind of intuition, in gaining an insight into this logic. Stekel, admired for his intuition, maintained that " we can talk of an ' inner logic ' of the dream ". The apparently nonsensical bits of the dream he considers its most betraying and indefensible points, whose solution guides in finding the meaning of the dream. Here is an example from his *Advances in Dream-Interpretation* :

> **56.** I climb a steep mountain. Two parallel paths lead up it. In places the path is swampy and slippery. A fence bars the way. A young man in an overcoat, with a bag in his hand, jumps the fence quickly and nimbly, while I, who have neither overcoat nor bag, surmount the obstacle only with great difficulty.

" From previous dreams of the patient it appeared that *bags signified for him marriage, while the overcoat signified the warming and protecting nearness of the wife.* The dream urges the dreamer to

[1] Cf. p. 196.

marry : a married man is better protected than an unmarried one, against the temptations and difficulties of life (the *two* paths, the swamp, the fence). He is better able to surmount the obstacles of life."

(10) A lack of " real logic " is shown also by the so-called *condensation in the dream* (which will be dealt with at greater length in Ch. XII). A very interesting example of this phenomenon is the dream, which occurred to a man during a conflict-situation brought about by a love-affair :

> **57.** I have had no news from my girl-friend for a long time. She lives in America. In my dream I go there, but somehow I arrive at the house of another family. The house is not very attractive. I want to go to the post office to notify her of my arrival. Then I am again in an ugly room. Two beds in front of me are far apart, near the two side walls. An elderly woman and an elderly man lie in the beds. The woman is my mother, but also Mrs. Nutall. I don't know the man, perhaps he is Mr. Nutall, although actually he does *not* look like him. Perhaps it is *I* who am lying in the bed, with a funny little hat on. But at the same time I am standing between the two beds ; an ugly girl is in the room ; at the same time I see my beloved in my imagination.

Associations of the dreamer : " I remember how, as a child, I happened to enter into the poor house of an old couple ; they had been married only a few hours previously (both had been widowed) and were just about to go to bed. I wondered whether people of their age still had sexual desires. . . ." In connection with the man in the bed, he remembered a doctor, whose practice was very successful financially, but who used to wear a *small* old hat ; his wife looked a trifle elderly, but very pleasant. Also, he remembered another doctor, a widower whose marriage was not very successful ; further, a pale, thin labourer whom he met during a voyage, and of whom he knew that he was a bachelor and lived with his mother. This man had gastric trouble and was anæmic (so was also the dreamer at the time of the analysis). This working class man seemed to resemble the figure in the dream more closely than any of the other people mentioned. . . . In order to understand the dream we must add that the dreamer wants to end his own unsatisfactory conditions at home, and to marry his girl-friend. But in order to do that he would have to be rich, like the doctor in the associations ! In this conflict-situation he undergoes an *infantile regression, his libido returns*

to the mother-fixation, from which he suffered up to the age of 25.
(See the working man in the associations.) His mother and
Mrs. N. in the dream have *one* thing in common ; according
to the dreamer they were both frigid and lived only for their
children ; hence they succeeded in bearing their widowhood
well, in spite of financial difficulties. *The comical male figure
in the dream, then, represents the patient and his mother-regression ;
also his feeling of being old* (like the elderly couple). This
identity is well supported by the associations ; also there was
in the dream the appropriate *feeling of identification.*

This whole example demonstrates clearly how all the details
of the dream represent deep psychic contents, parts of the ego,
and how the phenomenon, called *condensation*, is fundamentally
nothing but intensive and abundant dramatisation and personification of the dreamer's subjective state. There is no difference in principle whether the ego appears in the dream split
up in its various tendencies, and represented by different
persons, actions, things or localities, or whether, on the other
hand and reversely, a certain psychic constellation in its unity
is being represented by a homogeneous scene in the dream,
the latter consisting of several super-imposed images, which
are woven into a unity.

De-composition (dissociation) and condensation [1] *in the dream are
two forms of ego-dramatisation.* At any rate there is, as we have
seen, a simple explanation for a characteristic property of the
dream, a property so different from the logic of waking thinking, i.e., the simultaneous superposition of elements of a
different kind, and belonging to different historical levels,
without any objection by the dream-ego towards such " real
impossibility ".

(11) One can experience fully this feeling of " natural
acceptance " of unreal events in the dream, only within one's
own dreaming. An experienced analyst said : " I remember
only few such dream-situations from my own experience ; but
I remember very vividly the accompanying feeling of absolute
natural ' self-evidence '. It was always an intensive adventure
for me to live through the multiplicity of events in such a
complicated and illogical dream. Compared with waking life,
the latter seemed almost drab, monotonous and poverty-
stricken. True, even in waking life I have no difficulty in
experiencing the polyphony of my thinking process, and I can

[1] Cf. Ch. XII (1), (2).

pursue two trains of thought at the same time with ease ; write or read *and* listen to a conversation. Thus I have a certain conscious sense of how these things happen in the dream. I never view the illogical jumble of my dreams after awakening with such a feeling of surprise as other people do, who have not been analysed and whose thought proceeds only on *one*, clear-cut level."

We have pointed out that the dream-events constitute an *experience*. We must lay stress on the fact that dreaming itself, quite apart from the particular dream-image, is an experiential process. In waking thought, too, we can distinguish clearly the *process of thinking* from the content and subjects of it. In looking for a rough analogy, the present author used to refer to an escalator ; the escalator in movement, and the people who may be using it, are quite separate entities—the stairs move whether anyone boards them or not. Similarly with the dream-process and the psychosomatic material which is transformed and shaped into the dream-experience. But in dreaming there is never a state of " emptiness " ; only a lack in formed conceptual material. *This corresponds perhaps with the state of perfectly dreamless deep sleep.* Stekel, indeed, went so far as to maintain that we dream continuously, even in the waking state ; that in the background of the thinking process the co-conscious, and subconscious stream of " dream-phantasies " passes by without interruption. Our waking thought, accordingly, would be *polyphonous*, after the manner of a well-instrumented orchestral piece, which contains the middle parts and the counterpoint, in addition to the leading melody. Day-dreaming proper is, according to this author, a sign that the former levels have gained the upper hand. As he maintained in his *Störungen des Trieb und Affektlebens*, Vol. VIII : [1] " In neurotic fits of unconsciousness, as well as in sleep, the affect-cathexis of the middle parts and of the counterpoint becomes stronger than that of the leading melody." He believed also that " a complex day-dream process precedes the final verbalisation of our thoughts ". " Words are, in fact, final compromise-formations, resulting from the struggle of different trends of thought." We fully agree with this conception. However, it is easy to see that waking thought strives for " form " ; and accordingly the " dreams " of waking thought are " formed " entities. In deep sleep, on the other hand, the " unformed "

[1] *Sadism and Masochism*, translated into English by Brinkle.

dreaming, an experience void of " formed " components in the sense of waking-thought, probably occupies the stage.

(12) Since the present author relates the dream and the dream-forming energetic material (dream stimuli in the old terminology), to the whole psychosomatic organisation, it follows that there must be *innate dream-contents, complexes and motifs*. Jung's conception [1] on this point constitutes essentially a postulate, which follows from our conception on dreaming formulated on lines of natural science. It is clear, for instance, that the element " motherliness " as the source of life in general, of individual being, and on the other hand the concrete mother figure as a love-giving and beloved object, belong to one and the same entity. This is similar to the explanations given above (8) that elements : stomach, desire, disgust, etc., form also a psychophysical unity. These considerations *may* at times, in individual cases, carry a practical importance in psychotherapy ; though mostly this seems not to be the case. Our whole organism is a unity (a viewpoint which has been recently stressed by all modern authors too frequently to need special mention), and it strives for restoration of this unity. This is also the case when the dream combines various sources into *one* unitary experience. Stimuli which cause us to awaken, in fact, exogenous stimuli in general, illustrate aptly this principle, by the manner in which they are becoming woven into the dream-action.

Someone is asleep in a garden. He dreams :

> **58.** Something interesting is about to happen. Some sort of discussion, but the two speakers are to debate in such a manner that each speaks alternate sentences. It strikes me as comical, like an opera with two singers, who declare their love for each other. . . .

On awakening, the dreamer heard two working men hammering a stone, pounding it with alternate blows. Sante de Sanctis also mentions this phenomenon, and deduces from it, that waking consciousness remains functionally operative *beside* the dream-consciousness ; as we can see, it remains capable during the dream of receiving stimuli from the outside and of transforming them. In the chapter on *Interpretation* we shall give a good example which also shows clearly that *fundamentally there is a tendency to bring about a unity, and illustrates how the*

---

[1] See also Ch. XI, p. 184, and XII (22).

exogenous impression takes on a psychic content.[1]   I may remind the reader of my hypothesis that all organic regions carry and develop a psychoaffective content [2] which they supply to the dream-work.   What we see in these unifying dreams, is fundamentally the same *tendency to furnish everything physical with a mental content.*   I might also refer to the section dealing with the " position of the body " in its influence on the dream-structure where the same aspect is dealt with.

[1] Cf. Ch. XII (15).   [2] Cf. Ch. V (5).

CHAPTER VI

FREUD'S THEORY OF DREAMS

(1) IN this chapter we shall try to give a brief but precise account of Freud's theory of dreams, which has been the foundation of all advances in this field. Even to-day, the great number of his closer followers look upon it as the only valid theory, sufficient in its every detail. Freud distinguishes (1) the manifest dream, i.e., the remembered, verbalised description of the dream ; (2) the latent dream-thoughts, i.e., the supplements to, and sources of, the various parts of the dream, brought to light by means of free association and interpretation ; (3) the actual dream stimulus. *This last factor is always a wish-tendency.* As one can see from a careful scrutiny of Freud's writings, it is an *unconscious wish* ; an instinctive drive, originating in infantile sexuality, which has suffered repression, but which has always remained active. This drive supplies the *energy* which combines with various thoughts, memories, etc., and constructs the manifest dream. The elements are *transformed symbolically* to varying degrees. One of these elements called the " day-residue ", is a recent memory from the day before the dream. " The pressure of the unconscious wish on the day-residue creates an additional part of latent dream-thoughts " (*Introductory Lectures*); in other words, the latter become connected with the former energetically charged element. The whole formation is a hallucinatory experience whose psychic value lies in the satisfaction of the latent wish. *The wish-fulfilment, as the final result from the sub-jective point of view of the dreamer, would thus represent the fourth factor of this dream-theory.* In Freud's larger work on dreams he constantly emphasises, however, that the wish which is becom-ing fulfilled in the dream, is not always a sexual one, and that the dream also fulfils other wishes of the dreamer. But in the final analysis of his writings it remains true that for Freud the *fundamental cause of adult dreaming is infantile sexuality*, which combines with elements of a different kind, and so, too, with different wishes of recent actuality. That particular agency which initiated the original repression and which maintains it by means of a " counter-cathexis ", is responsible also for the

disguising of the wish-fulfilment, effectuated by the dream-work. Indeed, it is only the weakening of this " censor " during sleep, which makes it possible for the infantile wish to become sufficiently active, to stimulate dreaming, and to construct the dream-image by means of the latent thoughts. Freud calls the retreat into sleep a *regression* (to the infantile or even to the pre-natal). The re-animation of the infantile wishes in sleep is a consequence of this regression, or rather *one* aspect of it. Freud regards also the representation through symbols and visual images as regressive ; first he reduces the *symbols* to *archaic modes of speaking and thinking* (phylogenetic regression) ; further he believes that certain logical operations of the mind, such as causal relations, judgments, identifications, etc., can be expressed by the dream-ego only in a primitive way, i.e., by juxtaposition and succession of individual images. " After the manner of a primitive language only the raw material is expressed, abstract notions are reduced to their concrete foundations. . . . The representation of certain objects and events by means of symbols, which have become foreign to the conscious way of thinking corresponds both to the archaic regression of the psychic apparatus, and to the requirements of the dream-censor." (*New Introductory Lectures.*)

In view of the fact that the embarrassing character of many dreams is so óbvious, Freud is forced to distinguish wish-dreams, punishment-dreams and anxiety-dreams.[1] The latter two kinds represent the reactions of the super-ego and are wish-fulfilments of this agency. Even the repressed infantile wishes are mostly associated with painful memories, which arose from the fear of punishment, from the threat accompanying the original prohibition. The coming to life of the infantile repressions awakens also these memories, and thus the *wish-fulfilment dream* is often associated with a subjective *anxiety feeling*. In the case of traumatic neuroses where the accident is being re-lived during sleep, the dreams always result in anxiety states. Here the dreaming has failed in its purpose. " *Thus dreaming must be looked upon rather as an attempt at wish-fulfilment* " (*ibid.*). " Closer analysis of the dream shows that a great number of dreams in whose manifest content obviously nothing erotic is to be found, can be proved by means of interpretation to be sexual wish-fulfilments, and that many thoughts which waking consciousness recognises as ' day-residues ',

[1] Cf. Ch. XII (21).

are represented in the dream *only* because of the energetic aid given them by repressed erotic wishes." (*On Dreams*, 1921.)

" As an explanation of this state of affairs . . . we may point to the fact that no other group of instinctive drives has been repressed to such an extent by the demands of education and civilisation as the sexual ; also to the fact that it is precisely these sexual drives which in most people succeed more easily than any others in evading the control of the highest mental functions. . . . Almost every civilised being has, at some point or other, retained the infantile phase of sexual life ; thus we understand why repressed infantile sexual desires constitute the strongest and most frequent driving force in the formation of dreams. . . . *The majority of dream-symbols serve to represent persons, parts or functions of the body which carry some erotic interest and significance ; the genitals in particular can be represented by a number of highly surprising symbols.* . . . There are symbols of universal validity, which one meets in the dreams of all dreamers, within one and the same nation or civilisation, and others which are only highly individual, created by each person for himself from his own experiences. Among the first-mentioned, we distinguish those whose aptness to the representation of sexual functions appears justified directly through the customary use of language (e.g., those which derive from agriculture, such as ' propagation ', ' seeds '), and those whose relation to sex seems to derive from the most ancient times and the darkest depths of the evolution of our concepts " (*ibid.*).

In his first Lectures Freud asks why symbolism in dreams deals mainly with sexual objects and relations, while the symbolism of myths, of fairy tales and of language is more complex. In his opinion much that nowadays signifies different non-sexual objects, was indeed originally related to sexual objects, and to the act of coition. " The philologist H. Sperber, from Upsala, has maintained that sexual needs played a great part in the origin and the further development of language. Sounds were first used as means of communication to call the sexual mate ; in the further development of the various verbal *roots* they accompanied the communal work of primeval man. Thus the word uttered during this common labour had two meanings : it signified the sexual act, as well as the kind of work which was put on a par with it. In time the word was dissociated from the sexual significance and its application confined to the respective work. In this way a number of verbal roots were formed, all of which have a sexual ancestry." If this theory is correct, it opens up, in Freud's opinion, a possibility for understanding dream-symbolism. We should so understand why the dream which has retained something of these ancient conditions, should have such an extraordinary number of sexual symbols. The symbolic relation would be simply a remnant of the old verbal identity.

(2) CRITICAL EVALUATION OF FREUD'S THEORY. Whatever attitude one may take towards this theory, it is hardly possible to deny it a certain magnificent completeness. (Cf. also Ch. VI (11).) However, the reduction of all concepts to the sexual could, I think, be derived and described in a simpler way. Inasmuch as all *becoming* and *happening* can be reduced to the *most important act of becoming*, copulation, pregnancy and birth, we can see that all concepts which refer to our multiform life can be associatively linked with these " fundamental concepts ". I do not fully subscribe to Freud's theory ; not because it is improbable, but because it considers only the rough structure of events. It will be obvious, however, from our account, why it is that Freud recognised sexual and family-symbols in particular, and why for him these symbols have such a fixed significance. For him the dream aims at fulfilling infantile complexes (œdipal and other incestuous desires, with which are closely associated the ideas of various members of the family, and also the concepts of birth and death) ; consequently it is only logical that the various symbols should be understood quite concretely as genitals, as coition, as the death of the interfering person. After all, for Freud the dream deals essentially with such concrete biological events. It is natural that an analysis, which is being continued for a sufficiently long time, will in the end penetrate to the infantile level ; it is equally natural that behind all the psychic elements which together form mental unity, the sexual aspect, too, is to be found. Whether one finds the Freudian mechanisms always, or only at rare intervals, depends upon how one carries out the psychoanalysis, and what one is looking for intentionally in the dream-elements. Freud maintained that dream-elements which contained sexual material in a symbolic form, were particularly resistive to free associations ; consequently these elments had to be interpreted at any rate symbolically and actively.[1] It is true that all which is suppressed and dis-

[1] Cf. Ch. III, p. 92.

guised will be divined only with difficulty. But even according to Freud the symbolic representation is not a mere product of repression, but it is only employed, utilised by this mechanism. However, if behind the dream-elements mentioned, there are those so strongly " tabooed " and repressed infantile wishes, which are even less capable of becoming conscious than many other proscribed wishes, which *do* find open expression in the dream (death wishes against close friends and relatives ; breaking of sexual and legal barriers, etc.), then the disguised and disguising dream-formation is intelligible. Also the lack of associations to such symbols becomes intelligible in this way.

Yet I suggest another explanation for this associative inhibition. It is more probable that the dream-elements in question contain, to a considerable degree, contents which are " *incapable of being thought* ", contents from the region of the *scs.* which are too " abstract ". The deep roots of our instinctual life are so widely ramified, their associated " conceptions " in the deepest layers, so much richer than the correlated conscious counterpart, that most of their contents are " incapable of being thought " in the manner of waking consciousness.[1] And these elements are perhaps also too much " *organic* ", to be capable of being clearly conceived. (Cf. p. 213. Ch. XII.) Of course, we operate in psychotherapy with elements of conscious thought. And when we interpret, for instance, a weapon or an instrument as the male genital, it is probable that we have touched at least part of the corresponding total complex ; but without having exhausted its content, its significance, and without having interpreted it in a full degree. With this reservation we must admit *the correctness of the fixed sexual symbolism as postulated by Freud.* Jung in his book on Transformations and Symbols of the Libido (*Psychology of The Unconscious*), extends similarly the contents of the complexes and symbols.

(3) However, Freud's symbols have found corroboration in several instances and fields. First and foremost in the languages of various peoples ; but also in the myths and fairy-tales of all times, and geographic regions, conceptions have been found corresponding with Freudian symbols. Rank's interesting and suggestive writings may be referred to in this connection. Again, further confirmation of Freud's teaching can be derived from the experimentally initiated symbolic transformations of

[1] Cf. Ch. I (7).

sexual concepts. First, Dr. Schröter [1] following a suggestion
by H. Swoboda, made a study of the phenomenon of symbolic
substitute-formation in hypnotically suggested dreams. In
one case the following suggestion was given : " You will dream
of a sexual intercourse with your friend, first in the *normal*
manner, then *abnormally*. You will forget this suggestion, and
then *dream about it symbolically*." This was the dream of the
female subject hypnotised :

> **59.** Sunday afternoon. I am expecting my friend, whose
> birthday we are going to celebrate together. He brings a
> *bottle of wine* wrapped in an *overcoat*. He asks me to take
> a glass ; I do so and *hold it up to his ; he pours*. I suddenly
> take fright, cry out and drop the glass, which breaks, spread-
> ing the wine all over the floor. I am very much annoyed
> because the carpet is quite spoiled. He consoles me : " I
> shall soon *mend* that. Give me another glass to pour into."
> I fetch another, into which he tries to pour cautiously from
> the remainder of the bottle. But when the first drop pours
> into the glass *he tears the bottle away*.

Remark. " The strange, voluptuous movements of the
dreamer, which are difficult to describe, clearly belong to the
latent content of the dream." (Quoted after Silberer.)

In another case, the suggestion was given to dream about
a homosexual intercourse, but the word *symbolic·* was not
mentioned. Yet, it was again only symbols which appeared
in the dream. (Bag, key, staircase.)

Mention must also be made of the experiments carried out
by Betlheim and Hartman on Korsakoff patients. They put
indecent pieces of writing before their patients, who in recount-
ing them, changed them in the direction of greater decency.
Here is one of their experimental stories : " *One* young girl
was walking about in the fields by herself, when a young man
came up to her, attacked her and threw her on the ground.
The girl fought back, but to no avail. The man lifted up her
frock and inserted his stiff penis into her vagina. After intercourse he left the girl, who was crying aloud, and fled." One
female patient reproduced this text in this manner : " *Two*
girls went up a staircase ; two boys went after them. They
then married the girls, because one of them was pregnant the
other went home." *Mounting a staircase* is a well-known
Freudian *symbol for coitus*. A female patient replaced the part
dealing with the stiff penis by : " put the *knife* into the *sheath* ".

Another patient substituted " *cigarette* " for the *genitals*. Replacing the one girl by two made it possible for one of the girls to remain intact ; this is a frequent method of disguise in the dream. (Quoted after Schilder : *Psychiatrie auf psychoanalytischer Grundlage.*)

There can be little doubt that the symbols which Freud considered as " constant " often *do* portray historical sexual scenes, so that here the fact of dream-symbolism is clearly demonstrable. The analyst is quite justified in looking on dreams regularly, also " with the eyes " of these symbols, in view of the great rôle which sexuality plays in the life of human beings. But we must insist that the same symbols may also cover different contents. Sometimes (though not very frequently) I found that certain elongated objects occurred in erection-dreams of my patients (lances, sticks, weapons), when it could be shown by associations that the scene, or the object under consideration represented at the same time a different kind of content. We may point to the elongated object in dream No. 30, which was also accompanied by a moderate erection.

(4) At this point we shall discuss a problem of interpretation which is not without importance, and which deals more deeply with the rôle and the significance of the overtly sexual scenes in dreams. It is well known that Adler, Jung and to some extent Bjerre, while depriving such scenes of their manifest sexual significance, interpreted them often " symbolically ". Thus Bjerre tells of a man who put an end to a sexual relationship, which had merely a physical basis, and who gave expression to his spiritual severance and condemnation of this relationship in the form of a homosexual dream. This was interpreted to imply that the heterosexual relationship in question was as disgusting, as foreign to his real self, as would have been a homosexual one. The interpreter emphasises that no homosexual tendencies existed in the dreamer, and that this interpretation was the only possible one. We may think as we like about an interpretation of this kind ; we may doubt it, we are hardly ever in a position to test its correctness. The same can be said of Adler's interpretation of the incest-complex as a " finalistic arrangement " to frighten away, and to protect oneself from normal sexual relations of whose consequences one is afraid. It is possible, undoubtedly, that cases of this kind do exist ; it is a fact that certain psychopathic individuals are

more inclined to the development of such Adlerian " complexes ", than are healthy individuals who can cope with all the real problems of life, sexual ones included.

I would like, however, to cite an example which I have studied very carefully, and which shows, at least, that the sexual images *must not* always be understood in their manifest form. A rather autistic man whom I was treating once, was afraid of marriage. He was tied to his family, whom he hated openly ; his actual sexual life was definitely *hetero*sexual. He once dreamed :

> **60.** I see two women having *homosexual intercourse*. One has a male genital and apologises to the other on this account. (Wakes up with a strong erection.)

On my simple question as to *who* had once made apologies because of his genitals, he answered promptly that *he himself* had always had an inferiority feeling because of the smallness of his genitals, and that he had apologised for that to his present girl-friend ; she had said that she was quite content. This dream occurred during a period of great resistance, which could have been analysed as a negative father-transference. Negative transference in this case meant a strong but suppressed positive transference, an interpretation which could be shown to be correct by the life-story of the patient and by his true deep-psychic attitude towards his father. Thus this dream signified the homosexual transference to the analyst, who was represented in the disguise of a woman. The patient added spontaneously that the genitals appearing in the dream, seemed to be familiar to him ; then he remembered the genitals of his father. But even apart from this interpretation, it is clear that *the one, manlike woman is the dreamer himself*; that he is dreaming about his own intensive, obsessional inferiority feeling, and about his difficulty of gaining a correct attitude towards women and people in general [1] ; *this* is shown and experienced in the dream in the form and frame of the abnormal homosexual relationship. I think that this interpretation was quite definitely in agreement with the established facts of his life history ; and thus, it seems to support the assumptions of the authors mentioned. This case has certainly convinced me of the possibility in principle, of their view ; it should, there-

---

[1] One could certainly reduce the lacking " social faculty " to some basic deficiencies in the " sexual organisation ". However, modern progress in analytical psychology does not permit such simplifications.

fore, certainly not be left out of account. In the present case the dream-genesis might be explained in this manner : When the libidinous tension rises, erection of the genital follows, accompanied by the formation of some dream or other. But at the same time the " inferiority-complex " related to this act is stirred, and joins itself to the sexual excitement and influences the dream-formation. It is from this angle that the psycho-therapist should look upon this dream-image.

(5) It is fundamentally impossible either to prove or to disprove the assertion that the infantile sexual wish constitutes the real energy-creating drive behind dreaming. If the whole psycho-affective life is formed by the libido, it may well be that dreaming, too, is an expression of this principle. Under no circumstances do the analytical method of association and the rules of symbolic interpretation give an obvious and cogent proof of this thesis. The chain of associations, as already mentioned, is, in fact, endless, and erotic elements are affectively strong enough to appear in it under any circumstances. What causes life, thought and feeling in general, is also the driving, creative force behind our dreaming. Is the fertilised cell a sex-cell ? The non-fertilised cell, yes, but the fertilised cell is already a living body. However, at the same time it *does* originate from the sex-cell, being a transformed product of it. Nevertheless, Freud's formulation seems to be too limited. Not incorrect ; not in the least in any sense improbable. It can hardly be doubted that the libido and its first individual forms are the seed, and thus the carrier of everything that originates from it in the course of life. But we dwell on safer ground if we ascribe the act of dreaming simply to the psyche, and also if we ascribe a more general biological function to dreaming.

(6) DAY-RESIDUES AND DREAMS OF ONE'S PROFESSION. We may add the following remarks with regard to the problem of day-residues. I have often noticed that there are great individual variations in the occurrence of dream-motifs, of items originating from the dreamer's profession. One might think that no other field would be more suitable for supplying the " day-residues ", declared by Freud to be inevitable parts of the dream. But as the present author pointed out once in a brief contribution (*Zum Problem der Tagesreste*, 1931),[1] this is true only of a few people ; others dream only rarely of their

[1] " A Contribution to the Problem of Day-residues."

daily work.   He himself dreams only at rare intervals of his
medical profession, and if, then usually about his work as
a psychoanalyst.   Kimmins, in his careful study of children,
confirms my own impressions, gained from adult analyses :
" Although the normal child spends nearly half the day in, or
associated with, the school, it is remarkable that so few dreams
have any direct reference to the school ; and where this is the
case, the reference is rather to the activities of the playground
and swimming-bath, than to those of the classroom. . . .
Indirectly the school has a great influence on the dream.   The
fairy-story has a very marked effect.   The teacher, moreover,
especially in girls' dreams, figures very prominently in dreams
of many out-of-school experiences."

Of course there are many occasions where important or
even unimportant memory-residues of the dreamer's professional life do appear in the dream ; particularly when these
elements deal with his own prestige, vanity, love, etc.   But
the specific " professional element " in the dream, particularly
when it appears frequently and regularly, has, in my experience, its " symbolic " significance.   I know that women who
are absorbed entirely in their household and their family, and
whose libidinous life is to all appearances rather neglected,
dream a good deal about their domestic duties.   I know of
one case (the mother of a patient), who used to dream frequently about soiled linen and washing, that is, about hard
work she had to carry out frequently.   Her son described her
as being quite disinterested in all pleasures.   Such cases make
it appear probable that the activity in question has taken over
the " libido " and the whole life-interest, and that it has
become in the dreams the symbolic representation of her
" everything ", a poor means of expression for all her endopsychic constellations.

In this way we gain also valuable insight into the phenomenon of " individual symbolism ".   I once treated a working
man of 35, who had suffered from impotence since the beginning of his active sexual life.   This man had only two kinds of
dream.   In a few cases he dreamed openly of coitus ; this
was during a period when he was told not to attempt any
intercourse.   Apart from these, he had *only* dreams dealing
with his job.   Not a single dream in its manifest content dealt
with his past, with his parents and other relatives, or with his
very numerous private problems which occupied him in his

childhood and youth. *It was quite evident that his profession-dreams gave expression to all these in a figurative, symbolic form.* (Cf. also Ch. III, p. 93.)

I would think that in this case the fact of his having been a total slave to his work from earliest youth, caused his dream-world to express itself in the terms of his job. I consider, as explained, the deep dream-processes as non-conceptual, and the conceptions expressing the dream-image as a secondary or parallel formation ; *one might say, as the first association pertaining to the primary deep dream experience.* In individuals of the above kind, ideas related to the work which holds them enslaved, offer themselves obtrusively as " *first associations* ". To give an example, here is the first dream reported by this patient :

61. The boss refuses to pay him for one afternoon when he, for reasons of bad health, did not work.

He said that nothing of the kind had ever happened, he had never been ill since he commenced working. What the dream gives as " not getting paid ", represents essentially that " which is missing in him ", i.e., it refers to his impotency. As far as the case could be explored (the therapeutic result came too quickly, after three months analysis) there was an educational suppression of his sexual development, which fact was increased by the hardship of his life, due to family conditions (step-father !), and additionally to different impressions which frightened him away from intentional sexual thinking, and activity. We might call this a " castration complex ", in a broader sense. It is very easy to understand why the poor man dreamed and produced free associations in apparent monotony continuously about his work and his boss ; yet, his analyst understood this language, and was so enabled to help him.

Another patient, who was a book-keeper, dreamt quite frequently about his book-keeping ; also all day long he thought about new methods of keeping books, although he was a failure in his professional life. I discovered that since he was 16 (he is now 50) he had kept an accurate record of all his pollutions and intercourses, for fear he might use up his energy overmuch. It was possible in this case, too, though only partly, to achieve a relief of his anxiety-states.[1]

Similar conditions prevailed in the dreams of a forty-five-year-old teacher, who could be relieved by six months' analysis

[1] Cf. pp. 11-12, the " Bluebeard " patient.

from his ejaculation præcox, from which he had suffered for twenty years, i.e., since the commencement of his married life. He constantly dreamed about school, headmasters, boards of directors, and about his *pupils* . . . until we unearthed quite straightforward incest-memories with his *brother* and *sister*, and an immense fear of his father at that time. After we had " worked up " these complexes, the number of " profession-dreams " decreased considerably, but still remained quite frequent. This man, too, was suffering from intense fear of loss of semen for 20 years.

(7) In my brief article on the relatively rare occurrence of professional elements in the dream, I felt justified in assuming that people who do not " love " their profession wholeheartedly, and who do not invest it with sufficient libido-interest, seldom dream about it. Where the choice of a profession is not an expression of the deep-psychic ego, of the personality, is not invested with the surplus of true instinctive energy, there is no libido-cathexis of the profession ; such cathexis would be more likely to take place with respect to a " hobby ". The examples given above prove, at least, the *obverse side* of this hypothesis, i.e., the frequent occurrence of " profession-dreams " when these professional elements *have* really attracted complexes and the life-interests. Now, however, this conception seems to me insufficient to explain the *non*-occurrence of such professional elements in the dream. I will now try to discuss the problem, briefly at least, from a different point of view.

Older authors have remarked that the dream often picks up ideas and problems which have *not* been dealt with fully by waking consciousness. Pötzl tried to find experimental support for this fact. He showed pictures full of colours and objects to his subjects for one-hundredth of a second.[1] It turned out that precisely those parts of the contours which were not perceived consciously, could be shown to occur in fragmentary form in the dreams of the following night ; those parts which were consciously perceived never appeared in the dreams. We may interpret this experiment in the following fashion : a psychic content pertaining to the field of our interests which is not " worked up " fully consciously, will be dealt with in the dream. Now, professional work, even if very interesting to us, goes along in an automatism, achieved through repetition and practice. There is little in it (apart from special tasks)

[1] *Experimental Dreams and Indirect Seeing.*

which is lacking mental adjustment, which is " unsaturated ". Only when the job, the profession, enslaves the ego, does it become significant, because in that case such activity is, for the deepest ego, " problematic ". Also, when the choice of profession touches or expresses a pathological complex (e.g., the sadist or the voyeur who becomes a medical man or a surgeon ; remember also the above-mentioned book-keeper, etc.), there ensues suitable dream-material. As explained in this work, I consider the dreaming-process as a function, contributing to the affect-metabolism. It is, therefore, natural that the automatically functioning job is least likely to undergo changes in its affective cathexis, and thus to employ the dream-process to a considerable extent. This conception, I think, explains the phenomenon fairly satisfactorily. Thus, we may take it as a rule that normal professional elements as day-residues will have only an *associative significance* for the dream-consciousness ; however, also the professional scenes in question themselves may touch directly upon some personal concern. But even if they do, in the latter case it is *not* the professional element as such, which carries the significance. It is true, of course, that one man will face his special profession, and the fact of his working in general, with more realism, and will take it more as a matter of course, than another, more given to a life of phantasy or of pleasure, who experiences every job merely as a " must ". Such differences might also produce differences in the frequency of " professional dream-elements ". I have been able to establish such type-influence quite definitely in several cases.

(8) WISH AND COMPENSATION. According to Freud, the dream serves to satisfy wishes, in particular those of infantile sexuality. Dynamically, hallucinatory dream-experience though disguised in formal content, is always a satisfaction, attempted or carried through. As Freud pointed out, the dreams of young children which are accessible for study, deal undisguisedly with the spheres of wishes, i.e., hopes and needs of everyday life. Kimmins says, in the chapter on " Dreams of children of eight to fourteen years of age " : " The number of clearly expressed fulfilled wishes differs considerably in boys' and girls' dreams, the percentage varying from about twenty-eight in the case of boys to forty-two in the case of girls." Freud, however, does not overlook terror-dreams ; these he explains as *punishment-dreams* just in connection with repressed

or proscribed wish-tendencies. It is obviously very difficult to disprove these statements. Admittedly, the critics have often misunderstood Freud and have dealt in their polemics mainly with the manifest content. But this much-debated infantile wish is supposed to be often undiscoverable, even in the latent thoughts. If one accepts Freud's ways and methods of proof, and the whole structure of his psychoanalytical theory, he will easily find also this wish-hypothesis acceptable.

Obvious wish-fulfilments, however, can be found abundantly in the dream openly, or recognised only by means of association. Let us look at this point more closely. In the first place, there are dreams which satisfy the desire to eat, drink, urinate, and so on, arising during sleep. It happens but rarely, of course, that the desire in question is being entirely satisfied in the dream. There is—as is well known—an attempt—often a repeated attempt—as the stimulation, growing more intense, remains. It is the eating-dreams (cf. below) where substantial fulfilment can sometimes be observed. The fulfilment of excretion-dreams is prevented largely by " social " consider- ations, which continue to function during sleep ; otherwise the hallucinatory experience of the incipient satisfaction might act on the sphincter muscle and lead to *real* satisfaction. Many bed-wetters really dream that they are visiting the w.c. Children who wet their bed occasionally also give this as an excuse.

Such social consideration does not apply in the case of hunger-dreams ; the dream-hallucination of eating can have only a good effect, i.e., the preservation of sleep. Coitus- dreams are not generally subject to such inhibitions either ; presumably because the " social " consequences of a pollution are not serious, it does not lead to such embarrassment. There are, of course, some individuals, who, from an exaggerated sense of cleanliness, force themselves to wake up, when pollution is imminent. Yet actually, for these people, sex in general is associated with ideas of inhibition. There is also another fundamental difference between the above-mentioned " need "- dreams and erotic dreams. The libidinous desire *does find* a great deal of relief by the dream, even if no pollution occurs ; while hunger and excretory needs can be satisfied fully only in *concrete* actuality ; and these urges inevitably gravitate towards such real satisfaction. Eating dreams constitute a certain exception here ; in this physiological sphere the *visual element* plays such a large part that the dream-hallucination can give a certain kind and degree of satisfaction, although not by any means to the same extent as in the erotic field.   In any case, sleep can be preserved by such feeding-dreams.   Since in the case of libidinous desires it is the psychic experience which constitutes the central source of satisfaction, the dream-experience can considerably, though not fully, replace a sexual event and its reality.   It is this point, too, which is fundamental for Freud's theory of dreams, which postulates the life-long dream-satisfaction of infantile desires.   The correct valuation of this fact will help us to view the wish-theory of dreams, in a more correct light.

(9) When a wish is fulfilled *in* the dream, then this is, in a certain sense, a concrete satisfaction.   This is perhaps too obvious to need lengthy discussion.   Not only has the dreamer the *feeling* of a concrete experience, but he *does* live through, in a certain sense, a real experience.   Day-dreams also may, in actual fact, compensate for the hardships of life.   I find it important to stress this fact in connection with another problem I now wish to consider.   The fact that a complex is being " realised " in the dream, does not mean that it corresponds with a " wish " ; not even with a " repressed wish ".   It is true that we say schematically, that the patient has repressed his proscribed desires into the subconscious ; for many cases and complexes, however, this is only a working hypothesis. More exactly : there are elements which are, *from the very beginning, destined only for the subconscious* ; elements which the psychic personality possesses, and wants to possess, but only *in a non-conscious form.   In these cases it is a realisation in the dream which is the goal, aimed at and wished for.*   In the sphere of waking wish-phantasies, too, we have a similar phenomenon.   We often imagine to ourselves situations which we enjoy *as* phantasies ; but whose actual realisation we would not at all welcome.   The sphere of phantasy is the desired field of experience.   The same applies to the world of " pathological complexes ", taking this expression to cover all those elements which *would* have to be repressed, *if* they were conscious.   We do not attempt to deny, of course, that in the dream real wishes of our waking life may at times be fulfilled, wishes for whose realisation in waking life we definitely crave.   In this latter case we are dealing with a *compensation*, a substitute-experience in the dream.   But those elements which the dreamer finds

strange upon awakening, which do not agree with his conscious strivings, belong exclusively *to the world of his scs. and to the world of dream-realisation.*

(10) Here we may mention a dream-mechanism postulated by Jung, and discussed in a lecture on " Die praktische Ver- wertbarkeit der Traumanalysen " in 1931.[1] He maintained that an *overstrong* positive sentiment towards someone (the much-beloved father, in the example he gave) might be com- pensated in the dream-world by the pictorial reflection of a negative attitude, i.e., by a disparagement. He thought that *both* attitudes were equally in accordance with the patient's " intention ", equally purposive ; that this was in a way a *regulative* and *compensating mechanism.* This assumption is attractive, and in its essence correct, I think.[2] Similar antag- onistic regulation can also be found in the world of the hor- mones. Indeed, this parallel may be more than a mere analogy, and may indicate causal relations. For, we may ask, what lies at the basis of such exaggerated " love-attitudes ", of such overstrong attachment and identification, when on the other side there is an inner need for damping them down ? It can be only the *neuro-hormonal apparatus* which effectuates the primary *over-reaction* (love, after all, is a psychic reaction, brought about by the influence of some other person on our own instinctive need for love). And surely it can be only the neuro-psychic organisation again which " counter-regulates ". The dream-image of the negative, disparaging attitude would then be merely the " personification ", image-expression of this inner counter-tendency.

The frequency of *openly-recognisable wish-dreams* (not in Freud's sense) varies considerably. My material, of course, implies experiences from more or less abnormal conditions. Nevertheless, I feel safe in saying that there are *several types of dreamers*, as is becoming more widely recognised nowadays. Different individuals behave differently, even in respect of wish-fulfilling dreams. The number of dreams which bring gain and not loss ; in which one meets friends and not persons

---

[1] Printed in *Modern Man in Search of a Soul* (Kegan Paul, 1933) (" Dream- analysis in its practical application ").

[2] I wrote once similarly in a different context :
" The overt resistance-dream may be interpreted as a first symptom of *the transference-situation.* It is an expression of the struggle against the submissive tendencies, against the emotional and libidinous transference, which latter would imply the exposure of the morbid ego to the therapeutic attack." (" Resistance- dreams " in *Fortschritte der Sexualwissenschaft und Psychoanalyse*, 1930.)

one does not like ; in which one enjoys oneself, and does not suffer ; in which one is the leader, or stands out in some other way, or at least comes up to an average, instead of appearing inferior, insufficient for the task, for his duty, is large in some cases, exceedingly small in others. This proportion is quite independent of the dreamer's real life circumstances. The wish-dream does not seem to constitute a psychic necessity to the same degree for everyone ; this is so in spite of the fact that the conscious wish for agreeable, successful experiences is quite universal. *The dream fulfils psychobiological needs, but not always wishes.*

ι (11) This law I discovered, quite independently, already at the beginning of my analytical practice.[1] Fundamentally, however, it was *Freud's instinctive-biological* approach which showed me the way. Although all those investigators who broke with the Freudian formulations have perhaps done more for medical practice proper than the master himself with his careful edifice ; only those who are familiar with the development of psychoanalysis know that it was the efforts of Stekel, Jung, Adler and others which led to the introduction of the clinically useful, more elastic form of dream-interpretation ; yet I am convinced today more firmly than ever that the greater part of Freud's ideas contains a correct nucleus somewhere or other, and will prove useful for the theory of our profession in its further development. I myself was unfamiliar for quite a long time with any of his writings except *Introductory Lectures*,[2] and see now with astonishment how so much of what has been discovered more recently is, at least implicitly, *suggested* in his works. Many of these newer ideas might have been only " co-conscious " for Freud.

As words express the thought-content, and at the same time narrow it down, so Freud's firmly constructed system (as long as it was not detoured by Stekel's personality, which breaks through rules and systems) did not allow foresight of the possibility of a shortened active psychoanalysis. And yet, behind the word, there is the infinite content. Similarly, behind Freud's rigid theoretical system there is a *wealth of yet unrealised facts*. They will be discovered slowly, once the philosophical

---

[1] See in " The Various Dreams of the Same Night ", 1931.
[2] As a young doctor, working for years in clinics, I was entirely satisfied by the *practical* books of Stekel ; although the author in the capacity as teacher, left his pupils full freedom in research. Somehow, only *very late* did I feel the desire to be acquainted with other types of analytical literature.

and dogmatic differences have been resolved. I believe, too, that the philosophy and the *Weltanschauung* of Freud, as revealed implicitly and expressed explicitly in his writings, will not be accepted at *any* stage of our future culture-history. But I am just as convinced that there also exists some deeper content hidden behind his words, a content which the great man himself refused to let emerge into his consciousness. Why, I do not know. To enquire would seem to me to be lacking in tact, because unwarranted. For I do not believe that Freud's "instinctive materialism" can ever do any *serious* harm to the culture, to the spirit of mankind. Humanity, I imagine, will do as I did—and many others also—it will accept that which is instructive, proven, furthering to science, and let the rest of his thoughts stream through its own soul, i.e., giving them that ethical and spiritual content which, in fact, is due to them.

CHAPTER VII

FOOD DREAMS

(1) FREUD quotes in brief three reports of authors who tell of the dreams of people living under abnormal conditions.[1] The lack of food, drink, and of ordinary luxuries in general, among members of expeditions, led to dreams, in which well-laden tables, valleys rich in water, rolls of tobacco, etc., frequently occurred. He calls the occurrence of these dreams *a reversion to the infantile wish-type of childhood*. The preponderance of simple dreams of this kind in children, he attributes to the fact that there has not yet taken place a massive repression of sexual impulses as in the adult. It may be, however, preferably formulated in a more general way, that the mental life of children on the whole is simpler, less burdened with problems and conflicts, and consequently so are their dreams. But where pathological conditions obtain, the dream-world of the child is also accordingly different. It must be borne in mind, however, that the child is not readily capable of reproducing, and probably of even remembering, complicated psychic contents. It is therefore never quite certain that there are no dreams of a more complicated nature.

A much experienced author writes with regard to the food-dreams of children : " The fact that very young children dream far less about food than older children, indicates that they are the last to suffer in the case of food shortage in the home. The dream is a sure indication of the position of the child in this respect, as is clearly shown by comparison of the proportion of food-dreams among children in poor and well-to-do districts. The child who dreams frequently about food may reasonably be assumed to be the *underfed* child. . . . The eating element in dreams falls off after the age of ten and the receiving of presents other than food, increase after this age. Dreams of presents and eating at all ages from nine to fourteen, are much more common with children from the poorer, than from those in the more well-to-do districts. . . . A well-known investigator was carrying on a research on the physiological effects of a short period of starvation. He remained

---

[1] Ch. III, " Dream as Wish-fulfilment ".

without food for six days and after the first day was not conscious of any personal inconvenience, but every night he dreamed of having hearty meals, though he had never experienced this type of dream before. On resuming his normal life the food dreams ceased. . . ." (C. W. Kimmins, *Children's Dreams.*)

Individuals who, like the above-mentioned members of expeditions are exposed to severe deprivations, do not necessarily cease to be adults ; they continue to bear their previous share of mental complexes. This type of manifest dream might perhaps be looked upon rather as a layer over the remainder of their dream-world, which latter has been damped down in intensity and put into the background of the dreaming-process. There appears a similarity to the organically stimulated dreams, such as are, for instance, the heart-attack dreams, which latter are relatively short, poor in scenery, and of a simpler structure. This indicates that the most pressing life-need in the centre of ego-perception takes precedence over everything else.

One might almost be tempted to give full agreement to Freud's sexual-genetic dream-theory, when one sees how in such states of hunger and deprivation these self-preserving instincts dominate the dream-world. What we mean is as follows : It is well known that in hunger and similarly in grave phases of several illnesses, the sexual instinct is manifest only in a weakened degree, or it is present only in a latent, inactive form. Thus, it seems as if the dream would grant satisfaction to *that* particular instinctive wish whose need was at the moment most stressed. The dreams of the above-mentioned kind might indicate that the fulfilment of the nutritional instinct in the manifest dream, has entered the foreground, because in fact, the libidinous forces are in abeyance. Yet, this conclusion is not quite cogent. As the same records show, various other matters, apart from the themes mentioned, occurred in these dreams. The overriding of everything else by the most actual and pressing life problem, appears, in the cases just discussed, all the more intelligible as the lack of elementary luxury, which has become in the course of life habitual, comes near to a true " life-threat ".

It has been pointed out in another connection that a certain real satisfaction accrues from the visual, hallucinatory *eating-experience* in the dream. This satisfaction value is definitely higher than, for instance, that of the dream-satisfaction of an ambition or revenge, just because the visual factor plays an important physiological rôle in the enjoyment of food in reality. We might add another idea, which has also been discussed in a previous chapter. We have spoken of the psychoaffective content of the various organ functions. It is very probable that the visual æsthetic enjoyment, associated with the food instinct, corresponds with, and fulfils, a relatively (though not absolutely) important biological need, which gains in significance and becomes stronger with the advancement towards higher stages of individual refinement. This need might indeed find a certain satisfaction by the dream-hallucination ; and so the compensatory value of the food-dream would appear still better explained. This satisfaction would lie accordingly primarily in the psychoaffective spheres corresponding to the physiological act of feeding. It is as if the organism could, to overcome the lack of nourishment, make greater use of a factor which, as a rule, is only a subordinate part of the total feeding complex.

In principle, however, it must be assumed that even such dreams show close associations to the psychic inner world, and—purely theoretically—there is no true reason to treat them differently from other dreams. For if, as we shall attempt to prove later on, dreaming ranks among those functions which satisfy corresponding biological needs, and if the material of the dream-image originates from the psycho-affective spheres of the individual, then, in fact, there is no line of demarcation between the various dream-sources ; and so the close relation with the affective world of the individual is a self-evident fact to be assumed with regard to every dream.[1] Here is an instance :

> 62. I am hungry ; my step-mother brings me some pastries. I don't know if *she* likes them.

The interpretable contents of this dream seem to be quite manifest without further explanations ; the bearing upon the private life of the dreamer is obvious.

The present author can confirm from his own experience that in his occasional food-dreams, which occur to him only when suffering from indigestion, stimulate regularly and without difficulty three associations connected with his father.

[1] Cf. Ch. X (2).

Identification with him played an important rôle for a long time. In the last years of his life, he was suffering from gastritis ; and the positive sentiment of the dreamer towards the sick man became intensified by the need of nursing him ; yet analytical frankness requires the admission that probably in consequence of the burdens of this nursing, which made necessary staying up at nights, some irritability due to fatigue, revived traces of an old Œdipus Complex, known to the author and dreamer of the mentioned dreams only through his training analysis.

There are no dreams which are not filled with psychoaffective material ; and this is so because there are no organic processes which do not contain affective elements as their inseparable contents (organ libido as the older psychoanalytic terminology would call it), and no stages in the course of physiological functions without having their psychoaffective counterpart. It should be therefore emphasised, that in our opinion the organically stimulated dreams when submitted to analysis, do not *merely awaken associations.* As Jung remarked once ironically in a lecture, in a different context, even a street-sign, or any inscription on a plate, might stimulate free associations, which in the end might lead to one's own complexes. What we want to stress is the intrinsic psychoaffective content immanent in, and produced by, the respective organic events themselves. The other associations thus are attached to a genuine psychoaffective element ; i.e., when free associations are produced to an organ-sensation dream, the former are stimulated not merely by the manifest dream motifs, but by the latent psychoaffective content of the respective dream, originating from the psychoaffective cathexis of the organic function which stimulated the dream.[1]

I understand from a fully documented article by Hitschman reporting on the dream-problem, that Alexander has carried out a statistical analysis of the dreams of sufferers from gastric disorders. " The analyses of these patients showed a predominance of dreams and associations dealing with nourishment, eating and drinking, i.e. *oral material.* Alexander and Wilson have naturally extended their studies to the oral tendencies which appear in the latent content. They found confirmation of their theory that lack of oral satisfaction was responsible for the over-activity and acid-condition of the

[1] Cf. Ch. V.

stomach. The objection that the dreams might be a *consequence* of the organic stimulation does not hold ; ample evidence shows that such oral dreams are the expression of oral-receptive wishes, which àre independent of the ulcer and precedes their development in time." [1] The present author is not very familiar with the field of " oral " tendencies ; he admits that he has never looked at the question through the eyes of the orthodox psychoanalyst. But he could, for instance, confirm from a few observations, that chronic " self-forcing " by overcoming feelings of disgust for a long time, by the necessity of eating food which is repulsive to him, or taking his meals in an environment unpleasant to the eater, can readily lead to the development of even organic disturbances. That means, that stimulation of a complex pertaining inherently to a certain organic region or a functional field, can, certainly, in some individuals, disturb the local circulation and cause injury. The observations of Cushing showing the aetiological rôle of hypothalamic centres for the genesis of gastric ulcers are well known, and present, in fact, some support for the theory of a possible psychogenesis of such troubles.

[1] " Beiträge zu einer Psychopathologie des Traumes ", II. *Internat. Zeitschrift für Psychoanalyse*, 3, 1935. (Contributions to a Psychopathology of Dreams.)

CHAPTER VIII

EXPERIMENTAL DREAMS

(1) I WOULD like to add a few comments on *experimental dreams* and their evidential value. I shall refer to three sources in the literature, and also mention some experiments of my own. Schrötter's experiments constitute the centrum of these investigations. He hypnotised his subjects, and suggested to them that they would dream. " In a few minutes they began to dream. The length of the dream could be measured because, according to instructions, they indicated the beginning and end of the dream by signs. After awakening they reported the content of the dream. In another experimental series the subjects dreamt during the night following the suggestion. In all these dreams the suggested element appeared to be aptly fitted into the dream scenery. For instance, the suggestion was : ' You have toothache, and a moderate urge to urinate. Within five minutes you will dream something ' ". The resulting dream :

> 63. We are in the *Prater* (an amusement park in Vienna) and near the " Watschmann " [1] (a figure whose ears one boxes, while the strength of the blow is shown on a scale). I hit him so often that his face gets bigger and bigger. Then we take a boat and row to an inn where we drink a good deal.

" The relation to the toothache (swollen face) is obvious, and the boat and the drinking point to the urge to urinate." The representation of the toothache is less disguised than that of the urinary stimulus, which is only alluded to by more remote associations. A genuine " organic urinary-stimulus ", as we know from experience, is usually represented more forcibly and overtly in the dreams. Of course, we can produce also a genuine urination-stimulus under hypnosis ; then, however, the whole state of affairs is different, because the stimulus is in fact, *a stronger one*. I believe, nevertheless, that there is no need, in principle, to assume a difference between the two cases. The idea of a " urination-stimulus " must be reflectorily

---

[1] A registering punchball.

associated with the " body-image " of the organ in question,[1] and the " psychoaffective charge " of the idea of urination will, particularly under hypnosis, reach also, in fact, the physiological pathways of the corresponding function, though only to a small degree.

Just as the endopsychic perception of the individual organ plays its part in the fully constructed " body-scheme ", so on the other hand, every affectively coloured " dynamic " imagination of the organ reacts on the corresponding peripheral regions. The reader's attention may be drawn to the conspicuous results of the autogenous training of Schultz, where the " experiencing " of one's own arm causes hyperæmia and warmth in it ; and the concentrated imagination of the heart stimulates certain, individually different, sensations within the circulatory apparatus ; a fact which was found to possess therapeutic value.

But in our experimental case, we should be careful to distinguish from this effect of " organic realisation " of the suggestion, the other part of the suggestion, viz., " to dream ". We have to distinguish three components within the whole procedure : (1) the production of the hallucinatory organic sensation ; (2) the stimulation to dream ; (3) the suggestion to dream about the sensation in question. This brings us to the point which is theoretically most important in connection with such experiments. The suggestion *to dream* mobilises the dreaming-process, in so far as it can be mobilised. We take it for granted that dreaming, of a non-conscious quality,

[1] According to Head and Schilder, the parieto-occipital transition region of the cortex is related to that function which results in the normal " self-perception " of our detailed body structure (body-scheme). We think, too, in agreement with Schilder, that from this cerebral region centrifugal influences upon the peripheral functions take their origin. We would not be surprised, if we learnt one day, that the normal dreaming function (as conceived in Chs. X and XI) is dependent on the intactness of this cortical region, more exactly on the interaction of this body-scheme centre and the thalamic-hypothalamic centres.

The self-perception of the body naturally reflects also the condition and state of the organs and body-parts as influenced by external stimuli. *In the " body scheme ", therefore, allo-psyche and somato-psyche coalesce into a unity.* This fact means that, as we stated, external impressions, perceptions become in fact ego-constituents. And all this implies the substitute-symbolisation of ego-functions and ego-parts by means of externalising dramatisation and personification. The mutual symbolic substitution of different body-regions appears also more intelligible since the different regions are parts of the compound, unified body-picture.

According to Schilder, the " body-scheme " consist even of different historical layers, containing the deposit of different life-periods. This, again, corresponds in some way with that mode of dream-formation which represents a present, actual condition by reference to some past memory and vice versa. I am aware of the vague, hypothetical character of these remarks.

goes on continuously even during waking, and quite definitely so during sleep ; this latter assumption was also made by de Sanctis, although not on psychoanalytic grounds. The suggested idea is then introduced by means of hypnosis into the dream-process, which runs autochthonously, and which perceives it, connects it with associations, and transforms it. The latter process is similar to the differential, transformed perception by the sleep-ego of mild sensory stimuli, which do not lead to awakening. (I am, of course, assuming here deep somnambulistic hypnosis.)

There is certainly a strange difference. When we suggest, " You feel a urination urge ", then the organic region will carry out the order quite plainly. But if the suggestion runs, " You have to dream about a urination urge," then the result is something different, viz., a hallucinatory dream-experience. The above hypnotised person knew, of course, that he was not supposed to feel any real urge ; that there was only a question of dreaming about it. Hence, only the pictorial, dreamlike representation. The fact that a suggestion of this kind comes into the dream only in a figurative, indirect form, proves the transformation of psychic elements in the subconsciousness. It may be, that the dream-representation in such experiments is indirect, pictorial, due to the weakening effect of social considerations, at work under hypnosis too (fear of creating a genuine desire and its consequences) ; or it may be, that actually a real though weak urge was created, yet it was perceived in a changed form owing to sleep. In any case, the fact that the dream-ego carries, and deals with, transformed elements of the *scs.*, is proven also by these hypnotic experiments. For, we have to stress that a genuine spontaneous, normally strong urge to urinate, as it is perceived during sleep by the half-awake ego, appears even in the dream as a more open, recognisable desire to urinate. What is even yet transformed in the latter case, is merely the *condition* of the dreamer, because this cannot be perceived in a real quality during sleep.[1]

Essentially, hypnotically suggested dreams are comparable to a dream, provoked or influenced by certain stimuli, as Maury applied them to sleeping individuals. He put, for instance, a hot iron near the face of a sleeper ; the following dream resulted :

[1] Cf. Ch. II.

64. Robbers entered the house and forced the inhabitants to hand over their money by making them put their feet in the hot *coal scuttle*. Then the duchess entered, whose secretary he was in the dream. . . .

I believe that the sensory stimulus influences the current affect-energetic dream, inasmuch as it changes the *secondary, conceptual level of the dream-image* in such a manner, as to make room for the sensory stimulus.

Thus the old question about the duration of the famous guillotine-dream [1] (which, although it was caused by the falling of a board on the neck of the sleeper, and which fact happened just before awakening, seemed to be very long and complicated in its antecedent parts) can be answered satisfactorily. The dream itself in its different parts had been going on for some time ; but its final, conceptual form (the secondary process), would presumably have been quite different, if the stimulus in question had *not* added the " decapitation " experience. I mean, that the *whole story* as it was remembered, would have been *quite different*. The stimulus exerted a substantial influence on the final conceptual form of all the dream-details, experienced *previous* to the stimulation.

(2) Hypnotic sleep leads to dreaming even without suggestion ; but these dreams belong to the group of the non-recollectable ones. This is at first merely a theoretical assumption ; we shall come back to it later. The suggested experimental dream is, then, artificially introduced and added to this dreaming. Naturally, the result is a compound structure, similar in quality to that due to the introduction of an organic stimulus into a current dream. But since the suggestion has focused the " mental vision " of the hypnotised person to the special suggested element, he will remember *primarily* those parts of the dream which relate to the suggested element and are connected with it.

I may refer here to what has been said in Ch. I, p. 15, that " unthinkable " elements may drag associated " thinkable " elements into forgetfulness. Actually, however, there is behind the suggested dream, another dreaming level. This may be deduced as probable from our explanations.

But I believe that in a suitable medium, traces of this " basic, background-dream " may be actually uncovered through deeper hypnosis, and by the suggestion to remember more

[1] Cf. " Freud Dream-Interpretation ", Chs. I and VI.

thoroughly. The faculty of recollection itself is, as is well known, facilitated by hypnosis ; and the reader might be reminded of the cathartic method of the first psychoanalytic period. I succeeded only once in carrying out quite satis-factorily such an experiment. Provided my experimental method is of a more general validity, it proves the existence of affect-energetic dreaming, i.e., of a dream which is not " think-able ". For, in two cases the medium reported, having felt and dreamt something, which could *not be remembered and expressed in words*. In one case, however, a colourful, muddled love-scene was played in a monologue, when the hypnotised patient was given the order to remember more deeply than usual. The dreamer was a woman under analysis because of depressions. She showed good transference, and she asked a few times to be hypnotised. First, of course, I refused ; but on one occasion I explained to her that there is nothing in the hypnosis dependent upon the hypnotiser, and that the actual realisation of such a state depended entirely on auto-suggestion. Thereupon she fell into a hypnotic state immedi-ately, and I made use of the occasion for the furtherance of the analysis. *No historical memories or intelligible free associations came to light ; but she produced fantastic dream-scenes.* One often finds that hysterically structured individuals reproduce under hypnosis concrete memories. In this particular case obviously a current " deep " experience, a dream-drama, was by word and action expressed under hypnosis. After awakening, there was almost complete amnesia.

I would not advise the employment of such a rather force-ful procedure in actual practice. Free associations to every fragment of a dream, or the artificial production of waking phantasies, will help the analysis along if there should be a halt in the dream-production. Stekel advised asking the patient to produce a short story, whatever it may be, i.e., an artificial dream. The method used by me accidentally in the above case constitutes a too vehement interference, which " fore-stalls " the analytic process and may prove a serious disturb-ance. However, in the above case, there was a strong desire on the part of the patient to fall into hypnosis.

At first, I had the impression that she was merely making use, half-consciously, of the auto-hypnosis, to declare her transference-love, without responsibility. As my understand-ing grew, I found the correct explanation and succeeded in getting similar, though not quite so complete, results from other subjects.

One might object of course, that it is not the non-conceptual basic dream which is brought to life under hypnosis, but some previously *formed* and even verbalised dream, which was, until the experimental moment, suppressed. I gained the impression, however, that in the mentioned case the whole material, which was produced in an explosive manner, was being formed *there and then*. We have to assume that in every analysis there is a constant, positive or negative, or bipolar, transference-affect, which constitutes the back-ground for the overt behaviour and speeches of the patient. This basic transference-emotion, and the assumed constant basic non-conceptual dream-process flow together during analysis. The conceptualised form of this was, according to my opinion, brought to the surface by the described experiment. The other two cases mentioned, reported only a *non-verbalisable experience* ; they too had received *no* special kind of suggestion, apart from the order, to remember the experiences through which they had lived under hypnosis.

(3) Silberer's " autosymbolic " experiments also contained an artificial factor, viz., that of the intentional self-observation. Everyone who carries out similar experiments on himself, observes himself, though unconsciously, but certainly, during the brief seconds or minutes as he is falling asleep, when the hypnagogic hallucinations are being formed. This implies, as far as I judge, that elements related to the *ego-function* receive more abundant dream-formulation than they would, if there was no " experimental attitude ". It was Freud who pointed out that we were dealing here with the same agency which, in other guises, acts as self-criticism, as introspection, or produces in psychoses the paranoid delusion of reference ; an agency which tends to become particularly strong in those " philosophically inclined ". In the type of experiment described by Silberer, the self-observation is, in fact, intensified ; this is the reason why these hypnagogic dreams regularly contain " autosymbolic representations ". The constantly current deep dream is displaced towards a back-ground, in favour of the observed autosymbolic element. (Similarly, as in the above mentioned urination dream, this element prevails because of the special attention.) This, however, means only that the autosymbolic dream-elements are formed less fre-

quently, when there is not such self-observation ; but it would be against all the rules of logic, *not* to assume that they are at any rate always present in the dream-process.   After all, fundamentally the dream deals altogether with the conditions of the ego, as it has been explained and supported by arguments ; and the mentioned autosymbolic phenomena are part of this ego-condition.

As already mentioned, it is often possible in the course of the analysis to obtain proof (through subsequent confirmation) that the dream-image not infrequently contains states of the psyche, purely abstract contents, and even sub-conscious philosophical conflicts.   Perhaps, there is an abnormal increase of self-observation and self-perception in all neurotic patients, which would explain the frequent formation of " functional contents " in almost every dream they have.   It is a fact that some patients fittingly interpret their dreams in this direction ; these patients were, in my observation, individuals whose whole thinking was in general increasingly speculative.[1]   But I want to express again my conviction that, fundamentally, the dream always contains also the functional aspect.   It would indeed be remarkable if this were not so, as everything that is represented in the dream contains and deals with the ego and its different individual relations.   We must not forget, too, that the person who is being analysed, is especially given to introspection to an increased degree ; hence the functional element in the dream is more or less furthered in its conceptual formation.

(4) Both Freud and Stekel pointed out that the dreams of the patient under analysis are frequently, and in an obvious manner, influenced by the views and explanations of his analyst ; the diagnostic value of such dreams is, therefore, questionable.   This observation is undoubtedly right.   However, I found that there are limits for such an extrinsic influence.   It is, for instance, difficult to stimulate easily dreams, in which the symptoms under treatment appear cured ; in which the agoraphobic can move freely, etc., if such behaviour in the dream was not the fact before the particular suggestion.[2]   Similarly, it is not possible to introduce into the dreams of the analysand every possible element.   The effectuation of such a stimulation depends obviously on certain conditions, and there must be surely an affinity to accept the particular

[1] Cf. pp. 36–7 and Ch. III (30), (31).   [2] Cf. Ch. XII (17).

suggestion and to deal with it within the dream-experience.

There is no doubt, according to my experiences, *that the dream does give, in certain cases, an answer of analytical significance, an answer to a question which was put by the analyst on the previous day.* I think that it is possible to induce a certain element into the dreams of the patient and to get the subconscious to deal with it, provided that the stimulation has not been carried out by the analyst in a challenging manner, arousing the resistance of the patient. According to a number of observations which I could make in the course of years, I am satisfied that there exists such a *complex-stimulation*, and that the reply given by the dream might prove useful, and further the treatment.

It proved especially useful to stimulate transference-dreams, since such dreams enable the conscious realisation of the transference, and of the possible sources of it. If, for instance, there is a substantial homosexual complex which is not being acknowledged by the patient, a suggestive stimulation will frequently make manifest this element in the dreams ; and according to my experiments, such a state of affairs proves useful for the smoother continuation of the analysis.[1]

[1] Cf. " Peculiarities and Problem of Dreams during Treatment ", I.

CHAPTER IX

THE ANALYTICAL SITUATION AS REVEALED IN THE DREAM-IMAGE AND IN THE ASSOCIATIONS [1]

(1) THE established close relation of the dream to the individual's intellectual and emotional life—both in its general causation and in its particular content—justifies us in regarding the dream-image psychoanalytically as a projection plan of the total depth-psychic happening. It is logical, therefore, to assume that an experience, so important for the individual, as a medical treatment, as psychotherapeutic intervention, in constituting an object of the endopsychic elaborative processes, will also emit its projections on to the dream-image. We find, in fact, both in the manifest and latent dream-content motifs, which obviously relate to the person of the analyst, to his private environment, his consulting-room, and last but not least, to his curative efforts proper.

> **65.** I am undressed ; my clothes are hanging on an armchair.

Association : The chair resembles that which the physician occupies during the analytical seance.

According to this supplement one can consider the "undressing" as having some bearing upon the "mental exhibiting" and expressing it in a symbolical fashion.

> **66.** I meet a friend of mine hurrying up the stairs.

Association : This friend suffers from heart-neurosis ; I think she was, too, *under your treatment.* . . .

Looking deeper into the problem, it is easy to realise that the analysis is not only *one* significant event of a recent actuality, amongst the other, different happenings in the life of the individual. The analysis embraces as its working object, the sum-total of mental life, experiences of the past, problems of the present, cares about the future, all feeling, thinking and striving, all that one hopes for or dreads. Accordingly the subconscious deposit of this broad analytical process is, in fact, congruent and adequate to the total of mental content. All the individual dream-elements during the analysis, therefore,

---

[1] Previously published in *Psychoanalytische Praxis*, 4, 1931.

are not only projections of the respective motifs, but at the same time representatives of the analytical process itself, in the reproductive and de-composing elaboration of which that particular motif finds itself.[1]

> **67.** I go towards my room with my friend. We come to the door, but I don't let her enter ; suddenly the door opens and my fiancé appears.

The patient feels that this girl might be a rival for the affection of her fiancé. This association might explain the dream superficially quite well, if we find in it the thought : " I don't let my rival come near my fiancé." When we add that in the subconscious of the patient there is a struggle between heterosexuality and homosexuality (as suggested by many other dreams and remarks), then we recognise clearly in the dream an allusion to this state of affairs, too, expressed in the antithesis : " Girl-friend outside, fiancé inside." In reference to the analytic situation, the dream-action must be understood in the following manner : " I go only up to a certain point with my analyst ; yet I do not allow him to penetrate in the depth of my true feelings in respect of my fiancé." Alternatively : " I myself do not feel like going into the depth of this problem."

One might speak of a *dream-condensation* of factual material and of the functional, analytical aspect. However, I would regard this rather as a working hypothesis. The following consideration might help us to come to a conception, approximating more closely the facts. Like all organic-processes, the dream as a biological phenomenon certainly relates to the present, not essentially to the past. Whatever points to the past in the dream, appears to have still some present importance for the subconscious, and to need the process of continuous assimilation ; this latter occurs, in fact, during the dream. In addition, the " endopsychic deposits " of past events, apart from their own significance, appear to remain in use as " thought-forms ", as " clichés ", as " building blocks " for any later eventuality in mental life and its deeper processes. Similarly, conscious thinking, judging and deciding occur automatically on the basis of past experiences—by means of " analogy-thinking ". In the dream, too, regarded as a projection of deep psychic events, everything relates in the first

[1] Cf. p. 192.

place to the present situation of the personality ; i.e., *we see in the various dream-allusions to past events analogies, symbols of the present situation.*

And because, as explained above, the fact of being analysed embraces the whole psychic status, we may look upon the whole dream, and upon every small detail of the dream-scene, as related to the actual analytical situation. There is no part of the psychic-content during treatment, which is not closely linked with the " constant " of " being an object of analytical elaboration ". The fact of the analysis is woven into the ordinary colourful and complicated deep-psychic event during the course of treatment. For this reason every product of the deep psychic happening carries with it the quality of " being analysed ", *and the dream as the projection plan of these happenings, mirrors in all its details the fact, the course, and the changing situation of the whole analytical process.*

(2) A young girl suffering from depression, dreamt after a few weeks of treatment :

> **68.** Someone reproached me because I used lipstick and rouge.

Associations : " The head of my department once told me that rouge would not suit me at all.—As a child I often looked pale ; my father used to ask why I was pale. To avoid this question, which was somehow embarrassing to me, and also to please my father, I used on such days to colour my lips and cheeks with moistened red paper."

The associations to the dream contain memories which seem to lend sufficient historical foundation to the dream-content. But there must be a motive, conditioned by the present, why this dream mirroring the mentioned recollections, has been dreamt at this point of the treatment. " Why do you disguise yourself, why do you take flight into illness, why do you refuse to see and to face the true cause of your depression, and to talk freely about it ? " It is this spontaneously emerging subconscious insight of the patient, that effectuates the allusion to that particular period of past in her present, by means of the cited dream. Another dream of the previous night ran like this :

> **69.** A lady I have known since I was a child reproached me for not having written to her. *I put forward my illness as an excuse, but she replies angrily :* " *How long will you go on upsetting your family in your hypocritical way ?* "

This dream, too, appears to originate in the deep psychic

recognition [1] being herself responsible for the outbreak of the repression ; of using it as a means to gain the loving care of the family, and of the father in particular. The associations in the previous dream, which led to the father, point clearly to this positive father-complex (" to please my father "). The present depression is meant to exert the same function as once did the rouge, to attract the attention of the father. To let this realisation penetrate, and not to show herself " in disguise " to the doctor also—that is the message of that part of the ego which strives conscientiously for health and fitness. It is to this deep tendency—as well as to the opposite one, i.e., still to colour and disguise herself—that the dream motif " to put on rouge " owes its present emergence. *Dream memories which originate in actual experiences and are being reproduced during analysis, serve as indications of the present analytical situation.*

(3) Although the sequence of memory-reproduction during analysis depends on the degree of repression of the various motifs (during analytical treatment these layers are being uncovered one after the other), we must also consider another factor. The actual analytical situation, the patient's degree of ability to reveal himself, the relation between the " tendency to be ill " and the " striving to be cured " on the other hand—these factors play their part in the selection of memories which are hinted at in the dream, and then more completely uncovered by free associations.

In ordinary life, too, a certain emotional condition is always accompanied by the presence, or emergence, of ideas and memories, which are adequate to that present state, either directly, or by way of contrast. Similarly, during the analytic stirring-up of memories at any particular moment, such ideas and recollections, as are in accord with the deep psychic and analytical situation, will enter the foreground of consciousness. We may give the following example : A young paranoid woman suffering from a mono-symptomatic persecutory delusion (" My cousin will poison me and interfere with my married life ") dreamt at an advanced stage of analysis : [2]

[1] The self-reproach might, of course, be a consequence of the depressive condition, and therefore not fully justified. Furthermore, I do not overlook the *hereditary basis* in this case ; yet this latter includes, too, a predisposition towards certain complexes. The *scs.* of such patients takes resort to these complexes when forming symptoms ; and the self-reproach in this particular case, might refer to the ready mobilisation of these complexes.

[2] A more detailed report on this case was published in *Psychotherapeutische Praxis,* 1936, 1.

70. I go into a shop to buy something. I propose to the proprietress that she might go to the tennis court with her sister ; during that time I will look after her business. While I am doing so, my young friend P. comes in, but somehow I am no longer in the shop. *We look for each other,* coming and going alternatively, but we *don't meet.* Dr. Lowy was also present.

Associations : " The proprietress of the shop has a flighty sister whose relationship with her husband was very bad ; she was supposed to have been unfaithful to him, and after his death she was living quite openly for her pleasure. As a child I had a girl-friend who was employed in that particular shop. I often took her place, and *sometimes stole some money.* I bought sweets with the money ; these I used to eat openly in front of the proprietress and my friend, and even offered them to the two women. Of course, no one knew where the sweets came from.—At that time I was walking out with a widowed engineer, whom I liked very much. My father did not like him, which only heightened his value for me.—My father never paid enough attention to me. *All his love went to my mother and my cousin.* (This is the woman who is supposed to persecute and to poison her.)—Mr. P. is a young man whom I like very much ; even when I became engaged, I spent a good deal of time with him."

The dream does not reproduce any direct memories, but rather constructs a new scene. Yet, it retains an illusion to the fact that in her youth the patient used to replace the sales-girl, which enabled her to *steal* the money. The latent meaning of the dream is that the patient wants to take the place of the shop-owner, i.e., *live for pleasure with her flighty sister.* (" To live with the sister " means also the homosexual complex.) Walking out with the engineer similarly signifies something *forbidden* because he was, in fact, an enemy of her father (and therefore all the more suitable to compensate the daughter for the love which her father has failed to give). The same holds for her relations with P. during her engagement period. The friendship with the former was carried on apparently almost under the eyes of her fiancé. (Just as the stolen money, or rather the sweets bought with the stolen money, were enjoyed in the presence of those who had suffered the loss.) *Thus, both the dream-content and the associations contain the motive " to enjoy forbidden fruits ".*

For analytic purposes [1] we may conclude from this dream that the patient recognises subconsciously the forbidden pleasure gain of her persecutory-delusion, and surmises her *loving interest in the woman who is supposed to persecute her*, and continues to relive again and again, behind the mask of her persecution-idea, the imagined relation between father and cousin and to participate in it as an onlooker. That the patient is really approaching deeper insight into the nature of her 'delusion, is revealed by the association dealing with her jealousy of father and cousin. This was the first time during the whole analysis, that the patient admitted *spontaneously* a positive, loving attitude towards her father ; up to then she had talked only of her antipathy to him. The dream, and the free associations to it, show the developing insight into the experiential nature of her illness. The patient feels that the libido has something to do with her persecutory delusion. If she now continues to cherish her ideas of persecution, *she robs* herself actually of the truth, and enjoys something forbidden ; something which her co-conscious has already recognised as forbidden, but which she cannot yet relinquish, due to a morbid compulsion. The identification in the dream with the shopowner (instead of with her flighty sister) also serves the purpose of disguise. The momentary incapacity to carry out the practical consequence of her endospychic insight (i.e., the abandonment of the persecutory ideas) is alluded to in the dream-scene : " We look for each other, coming and going alternatively, but we don't meet." The delusional idea and the original thought which was replaced by it (" my cousin's rivalry for the affection of my father poisons my nature ") cannot meet.

This example may serve to show clearly how the dream and the free associations and recollections connected with it, correspond with the deep-psychic situation of the moment, how they point to it, and how they give indirect expression to the analytic situation.

(4) The various associations which generally show no logical link with one another, are being produced under the pressure of a leading motif of the dream-content. This former in turn covers a deep-psychic dream-forming, affective complex. The chain of associations is, therefore, actually *influenced and directed by this dream-producing deep affective element.* Since the effect of

---

[1] I assume of course here, too, the primacy of the paranoid constitution ; the strength of the homosexual complex is a secondary fact, following from this constitution.

the endopsychic analytic situation finds expression in the manifest dream, the same must hold in respect of the chain of association. *The kind of associations also throws light on the deep-psychic state of the analytic situation ; and indeed everything the person analysed may say or do, is being dictated by the analytic affect, and consequently alludes to the attitude towards the analyst and his therapeutic effort.* We always think, speak, act and . . . dream in response to needs of the present situation, everything that is being remembered is only a symbol of a present wish, a present fear, *an expression of the present mental situation.* When, for instance, the person analysed recounts memories referring to the unfavourable outcome of various undertakings, or to unsuccessful medical treatments of himself or of others, we may be almost certain that his latent scepticism (or even the negative wish) with regard to the success of the present treatment is seeking expression. When, on the other hand, the manifest dream or the associations accompanying it, deal with a positive, successful attitude towards some respected or beloved person, then the reproduction of *these* memories in the dream, and the particular associations too, appear to be conditioned by the emotion of a *positive transference.* This way of looking at the dream-formation makes it unnecessary to interpret various persons appearing in the dream as symbolic representations of the analyst. *In whatever way a scene, involving motifs of love or friendship may be presented by the dream, this scene is, for affect-biological reasons, an expression of a positive transference.* There is no need to regard the various individual persons of the dream as mere substitutes ; *the dream reproduces and creates images which, in themselves, are adequate to the positive transference-emotion.*

> 71.   A man invites me for lunch, which is to consist of a great variety of dishes.   With some of these I am familiar, others are unknown to me.   I find it difficult to make up my mind, but the man embraces me, and I accept his invitation.

Associations: " My girl-friend often eats with us, and we go to the table *with arms linked.* She interests me almost more than my husband, who is in the habit of sitting taciturn. She also often helps me with the cooking, and invents dishes of which I never previously heard."

The analytic interpretation is obvious.   " However difficult I may find to agree with the solutions given by the analyst (variety of dishes) the interesting points of view and explanations he presents to me, fascinate me (the man embraces me). I have come to know a new . world (the unknown dishes), which, however, I actually have always carried in me —though hidden and repressed—(some of the dishes I am familiar with)." *The memory of the actual historical eating together with the inventive girl-friend thus becomes the symbolic expression for the analytic situation.*

The examples given in this chapter are of a relatively simple structure, which is not general ; yet they were chosen as illustrations precisely because of their simplicity. *I wanted to demonstrate the principle that the analysis-dreams and the free associations produced in connection with them, throw light on the analytic situation, i.e., on the most important question with which the psychotherapist has to be acquainted.* Everything else, the person analysed can talk about spontaneously, sooner or later. But he cannot tell about the finer day-to-day variations in the analytic situations ; because he himself is quite unaware of them. The only way by which they can be recognised is by the more penetrating interpretation of the manifest dream and the utilisation of associations.

CHAPTER X

THE BIOLOGICAL STATUS OF DREAMS, AND SOME CONTRIBUTIONS TO THE THEORY OF AFFECT [1]

(I) IT is proposed in this chapter to present a coherent description of some observations, established statements and theoretical conceptions about dreams. A life-phenomenon which is so very constant and general, pertaining so much to human existence, has to be considered as a *physiological process*, which is essential for normal life. The knowledge of all details concerning it, and also of all regularities and laws revealing themselves in this field, certainly merit the attention and interest of the medical world as much as other biological functions in man. Not least to be taken into account is that any theoretical progress, by extending and deepening our insight, might even pave the way to a certain therapeutic advance ; this aspect of our problem will be considered, though only in the way of brief suggestions, towards the end of these expositions. [2]

The dream-image, of which one becomes conscious after awakening, represents the result, the final product of the dreaming-process. This latter is, therefore, a notion to be distinguished from the dream-image, the former being *one of the functions of the psycho-nervous system*. [3] This concept implies the possibility of conceiving the dreaming-process, as taking place even when there is *no* resulting and recollected dream-image in consciousness after awakening. True, in spite of the impression that there was *no* conscious image proper at all, such might emerge during the later course of the day. There had still been, therefore, a dream-image produced, which had not attained that quality, in virtue of which the dream-image becomes conscious. There is, however, a kind of dream-experience, after which one feels during the half-sleeping state until the moment of awakening, that something definite and capable of being described had been dreamt ; yet after complete awakening, images and ideas, necessary for a " think-

---

[1] Reproduced from *Tijdschrift voor Psychologie*, Jaarg. VI, 1938.
[2] This concerns, in this case, disturbance of sleep.
[3] We do not identify, of course, *psyche* with the *nervous system*. We are, however, only concerned with looking at the dream-problem with, admittedly, a one-sided, biological bias. In Ch. XI a few supplementary remarks are added.

able " and coherent recollection, are absent, and any reproduction is rendered impossible.   The author holds that there
had not occurred any dream-forgetting ; that a forming of
images, in the sense of waking consciousness, had not taken
place at all, even during the dream-process.   We consider the
translation of the dream-feeling into the thought-forms of
waking state as a distinct and parallel, or subsequent, event ;
and in cases as these just mentioned, this transformation and
translation had not eventuated.[1]   There is, however, a definite
feeling, though no conceptual recollection, of a previous
dreaming-experience.   Such kind of dream-experiences present
a transition-stage to a further possibility, namely, that the
dreaming-process may occur without resulting in any conscious
final product, i.e., there does not remain even a vague feeling
of having dreamt.

It is possible to conclude approximately from the dream-
image as to the essential nature and function of the dreaming-
process.   The content of the former consist of : (1) elements
originating in life-experiences of the previous day and of the
immediate past (the day-residue of Freud) ; (2) elements
constituting deposits of more remote experiences ; (3) finally,
elements which cannot be easily referred to actual past experiences.   The recognisable elements, too, appear considerably
changed ; real events, or their parts, are being continued in the
dream ; or they are extended and modified in content.   At
any rate, *the dream-process is connected with the function of sensory
and mental experiencing.*

Since dreaming is so very closely and inseparably linked up
with sleeping, there is reason enough to assume *a priori* that
it has, more or less definitely, a relation to the assimilatory
processes of restoration and rebuilding in the cells, which
occur in an increased degree during sleep.

If we consider dreams which brought fulfilment to a wish,
denied by reality, or such types of dream which imply pleasant
hallucinatory experiences of any kind, we easily find in them
some indications of that assumed assimilatory and restoring
function and of the participation of dreaming in the general
tasks assigned to the sleeping state.

According to Freud—whose endeavour for systematism has
in any case to be acknowledged—the fundamental dream-
stimulating force comes from elementary, infantile drives, con-

---

[1] Cf. Ch. I.

sisting in libidinous, and jealous-hating tendencies which are directed towards near relatives. They suffer in the early stage of their manifestation a repression ; but after the fashion of non-fulfilled, because unfulfillable wishes, they retain an indestructible energy-cathexis, and they strive then constantly for hallucinatory satisfaction in the form of symbolical and disguised dream-experiences. Secondarily, also, wishes and problems of later, recent actuality are being included into the process of dream-formation. Essentially so the dream-process represents a means of wish-fulfilment. The proof of this doctrine with regard to dreams, lacking any trace of apparent wish-fulfilment in their manifest form, is of such a complicated and artificial nature that the strong opposition to this Freudian thesis is, at least, understandable. We want only to remark that complicated and even astonishing theories may still contain a nucleus of truth, though there may be a strong emotional reaction against them. At all events, the biological significance and rôle of these infantile tendencies has not yet been definitely clarified. Stekel, leaving the limits of the Freudian formula, showed that in dream the solution of recent conflicts and also that of the basic life-problem of the individual in general, is being attempted. This conception already suggested what the present author, extending the problem and considering it rather from the energetic aspect, formulated by the following statement : The dreaming-process is part of the biological mechanism including the total of affective events in a broader sense.

Anything which is considered and called from the viewpoint of meaningful, conceptual thinking, "intellectual function", is indissolubly linked with the production of affect. Any idea thought of, contains the combination of a conceptual element with affect-energy of a variable quantity. It is the latter which makes the purely theoretical concept an individually coloured thought, a mental element of personal significance, belonging to the "living" subject ; it is that which enables and effectuates the experiencing and "feeling" of the idea in question. *Affect is a " somatic " factor*, an energetic quality, bodily experienced ; any stronger affective outburst, emotional wave (of joy, anger or fear) doubtlessly runs and spreads throughout the body and is being felt by it. The total of human mental life implies, therefore, affect-energetic events.

The affect-energetic processes manifest themselves twofold ;

there is a purely subjective general emotional state (of joy, anger, fear, expectation, etc.) ; and distinguishably an alteration of individual organic functions, provoked by that emotional state, as palpitation, embarrassment of breathing, nausea, etc. It is, however, improbable that smaller degrees of such events should in their essence differ from the stronger and more obvious manifestations ; it is, therefore, logical to see in every, even the smallest, affective state, the similar bodily phenomenon. It is quite natural to assume also, that all such processes have an appropriate regulative mechanism ; and, in this sense, one may speak of affect-economy, of affect-energetic metabolism. This would imply the various affective currents, with all the parallel and subsequent organic changes. So it is obvious that one part-function of the neuro-hormonal system consists in the regulation of affect-economy.

What is called in general an emotional state, represents actually the stronger excitatory conditions and the more intense energetic changes. In fact, there exists also a continuous, more or less equally levelled, affect-current, besides the mentioned individual strong affective reactions. Similarly, the digestive process, gastro-enteral peristalsis, does not occur only at periods when there are subjectively felt and disturbingly strong single contractions. True, this is more a superficial analogy and external similarity ; however, we have to assume the existence of a constant affect-tonus, just as there is a stabile, basic muscular and nervous tonus. We understand by that a normal state of stimulation on a continuously equal level. The " emotional reactions " represent qualitative and quantitative changes of this basic, normal current.

The task assigned to the affect-regulative mechanism would consist in the " working up ", the elaboration of all kind of affects ; i.e., the utilisation of the optimal qualities and quantities, necessary or beneficial for the furthering of somato-psychic well-being, and in the possible neutralisation of affect-currents, undesirable and harmful in quantitative and qualitative respects. The necessity of such a regulation, and the probability of its actual existence, appear self-evident by the following considerations. The influence of stronger emotional conditions on the cardio-vascular, respiratory and alimentary systems is obvious. It is by no means justified and logical to assume, that affective stimulations of lesser degree gain no access to the same organic functions. It is also very probable that these minor affect-somatic events represent a factor, desirable and beneficial for life, for vigour, for the normal life-tonus. There must, therefore, exist an optimal condition, the excess of which is comparable to a hyper-hormonal flow and its consequences for physiological balance. It might be remembered that in the latter field also there is in operation an antagonistic and antihormonal regulative function, in order to maintain healthy conditions.

The dreaming-process, then, seems to be incorporated in this broader regulative mechanism. This is the proper and fuller meaning of what was briefly formulated earlier by the present author, that the dreaming-process serves the affect-economy and the affect-metabolism.[1] *One* of the conditions of sound sleep is the smooth course of the dreaming-process. This implies the efficient elaboration of the affect-energetic elements by the special way of the dreaming-act. Dream-situations leading to awakening, indicate that the dreaming-process has become strained, comparable to an overburdened stomach. Too intense peristalsis similarly disturbs the homo-geneity of the ego-feeling, both during waking and sleeping states. Since the final, conceptual dream-image which is being consciously remembered, is created in the state of superficial sleep, it is natural that any forcible awakening, brought about by such overburdening and disturbance of the affect-met-abolism, is being accompanied by an unpleasant dream-experience, mostly of the anxiety or disgust group. The latter, if not of vascular origin, indicate, therefore, difficulties or inefficiencies in the process of affect-elaboration in general, and perhaps not only the primary presence of genuine guilt and fear complexes actively at work. See, however, Ch. V, (7) and (8).

It is known that in the course of longer analytical treatments incidental sleep-disturbances improve, without any special suggestive interference to that end. The analytical process, in virtue of its specific dynamism, relieves the affect-economy, and effectuates artificially a considerable part of the affect-metabolism, i.e., it enables and facilitates a smoother course of that physiological process which normally occurs during sleep. An ideal hypnotic ought, therefore, to influence also the affect-energetic process, partly by damping down its tension, and partly by stimulating, furthering positively, its course.

---

[1] "The Various Dreams of the Same Night," 1931.

Investigations, considering this aspect, might to a certain degree improve the rational composition of sleeping-drugs.

(2) In view of the obvious fact that organic events (such as the peristalsis of the overloaded stomach, or a bronchitis impeding the breath, or toothache, or fever), exert an essential influence on the dream-formation—and this both with regard to its general affective colouring and its special content—it is customary to speak of somatic dream-stimuli and sources, in addition to the psychic, experiential ones. Such are the various unpleasant dream-experiences fraught with anxiety, disgust and initiated by different organ-disturbances ; the source of the stimulation being more or less hinted at by the special dream-content. Such are, for instance, dreams influenced by urinary urge, in which one looks for a toilette, or spills a glass of water ; or dreams with obvious erotic content, accompanying erection and pollution, which are formed on response to an increase of libidinal excitation.

There is a reasonable need for a unified conception of the total dreaming-process, which would consider the *two kinds* of dream-stimuli as having a *common* denominator. It is logically justified to assume that that energetic element, which is selected and perceived by the dream-process from psychic sources, is, in its essential quality, similar to those stimuli which are called the *somatic* ones. That means : a contraction of the intestines, subjectively felt, seems to contain, besides its pain character, an excitation-quality which, in subjective self-perception, appears similar to that of a psychogenic element. By this we want to assert that *organic functions imply, and also produce, affect-energetic qualities*. These affect-currents, originating from and running through the organs, constitute the so-called somatic dream-sources. There is much in favour of the idea that all the subjectively felt affective excitements, of various intensity and of variously gradated quality, experienced as emotion in the waking state, essentially consist in specific waves of stimulation of the organism, i.e., in specifically modified stimulations of its various parts. That which is experienced in joy, fear, expectation, and also that which accompanies the experiencing of any thought-content, relevant to the personality, and the total affect-tonus in general, originates in the periphery, in the organs. This part of the James-Lange theory, so far as the *final energetic current of the elaborated subjective emotional state* is concerned, seems, for the emotions of man, incontestable. It is, therefore, no wonder, that in sleep *also* reflections of organic events so frequently and considerably influence the dream-image and the dreaming-act. *In fact, this transformation of organic energy into an affective one, within the process of dreaming, seems to be a confirmation of the close relation between emotional experience in general on the one side, and specific peripheral excitations on the other.* It may be borne in mind that the dream theory of Scherner tried to deduce all dreaming and all dream-images from the normal and abnormal organic functions, assuming that all the dream events are essentially symbolic reflections of physiological processes. Freud, however, rightly notes that there is no purposive function of dreaming in the exposition of this author. One could gain the impression that " the psyche deals only playfully with the stimuli presented to it ". According to our new, modified conception, the affect-regulative mechanism, a branch of which is the nightly dreaming, has the task of elaborating and regulating *all* the affect-energetic qualities, the similar physical stimuli, coming *primarily* (i.e., not as a consequence of the emotions), and continuously, *from the organs* included. We do not think here merely of the abdominal or glandular organs, but to the same degree of muscles and skin. Thus, it is intelligible why all stimuli, impinging on the sleeper, produce dreams. These dreams are, in fact, merely signs of that process, which elaborates and assimilates the stimuli ; a process which, in a different quality and quantity, takes place also in the waking state. Naturally, the field of " organ-sensation dreams " has to be regarded as infinite ; *behind every dreaming there is the whole psychosomatic life-process.* The extent of the " organic dream-sources " is, therefore, far greater than is generally admitted by present-day psychologists of modern psychoanalytical orientation. Our conception assumes, in agreement with older authors, that the total of organic processes is a constant and substantial dream-source ; but it supplements this conception by taking into account at the same time the infinite wealth of the psychic sources and considering both kinds of dream stimuli as qualitatively similar.

All that has been said so far, enables us to believe, that the dreaming-process, which in the absence of waking consciousness results in the dream-images proper, continues operating even in the waking state. The assumed affect-metabolism, to which it is related, is similarly a constantly occurring process ;

as is the case in general, with all the other biological functions. The creating of dream-images during sleep is, therefore, only *one* partial function of the whole dreaming-process. That is why the present author suggested the consideration of the dream-image, which enters consciousness and waking memory, *as a final metabolic product of the total dreaming-process* ; or more exactly, of the affect-metabolic processes on the whole.[1] This idea, too, has its incomplete " forerunner " in the scientific literature. Robert [2] (1866) believed that dreams represent *excretions of thought-elements*, not having developed beyond their vague, initial embryonic form ; their accumulation, if not gaining vent, could be a source of mental disturbance.

Stekel, however, even asserts—and manifold experiences of practical psychoanalysis seem to confirm this—that even the formation of genuine images takes place constantly, i.e., even in waking, though only in an unconscious quality. *Day-dreamers* are individuals in whom such dream-formation, normally occurring only in the back-ground of consciousness, becomes intensified and encroaches on clear consciousness. *Obsessional thoughts* similarly represent day-dream elements, protruding with force into awareness and experienced by a part-ego as a kind of reality. *Delusions, delirious formations* in various psychotic states, and similarly those of intoxications, are also kinds of dream-experiences coming into being during waking state, and following the organic deterioration of the inhibitory barrier, they intrude into consciousness.[3]

The meaningfulness and the complicated structure of this metabolic end-product, i.e., of the dream-image, and also its value for depth-psychological research, is comparable to the essential significance of the other " material " metabolic end-products. Nevertheless, the dream-image possesses, at any rate, a far higher potency ; as dreaming itself means essentially more than a mere metabolic process. The meaningfulness of all psychic phenomena, the dream included, is an additional characteristic apart from their purposiveness.[4]

At any rate, the conception of Stekel already mentioned, according to which even genuine dream-images are created

---

[1] " *Psychotherapy of Paranoid Conditions*," 1932. Cf. also Ch. III, p. 95, and Ch. VI (7).
[2] Quoted by Freud.
[3] All these formations are, of course, different in many ways from the dream-image experienced during sleep. Common to all of them is the realistic, " concrete " experiencing of what is, in fact, but an intrapsychic element.   .
[4] Cf. Ch. XII, pp. 234–5.

N

in the waking-state, strengthens the probability of the assumed constant dream-energetic and affect regulative system. This inclusion of the dreaming-process into the group of the other biological processes necessary for normal life, enables us to reach a deeper realisation of both the overwhelming rôle of recreative sleep for mental well-being, and similarly the unfavourable influence of a disturbed night, especially on general mood and intellectual faculty. In sleep, which itself, according to modern research, represents an active, positive function of the psycho-nervous system and not merely a " negative rest ", the work of the affect regulative mechanism is intensified and extensified, as compared with the waking state.

The following interesting observation of daily life finds, too, its explanation on the lines of our conception. It occurs frequently that one is awakened from sleep by force, or by some sudden disturbance ; one, however, feels the intense need of a few minutes more sleep, in order to attain the satisfactory feeling of having slept enough. If this need for further, though short, sleep is not satisfied, the whole day might be disturbed. If, however, it has been granted fulfilment, the previous whole night's sleep attains *only then* its completion. I think, in such cases there is a yet unfinished dreaming-process, perhaps a particular dream-image has not yet been brought to completion, or something similar.[1] In no case is it a question of a simple " negative rest " and mere passivity of sleep, since in this respect such few minutes could hardly be of any substantial importance. Experience shows that on certain days one is more fit for work after a night of comparatively less sleep—if for instance the latter has begun later than usual— than on those days when one feels moody and miserable in consequence of such unsatisfied " last minutes " of sleep. Even such a brief period might be easily of substantial importance if it is a question of an undisturbed and uninterrupted rounding off of a dream-phase. Similarly, we know some individuals for whom a " nap " of one or two minutes enjoyed during the course of their work, suffices to restore mental and physical fitness. Dattner, in pointing to this observation, speaks of a " vegetative switching over " which occurs in such

---

[1] The falling asleep again, after having been almost awake, implies, of course, the re-starting of a new dreaming-phase, and makes the new attempt at active intentional awakening more difficult. (T. Hart.)

moments. We think that the essence of this phenomenon might also be explained satisfactorily from the viewpoint of affect metabolism which, as mentioned above, is more intense during sleeping and dreaming.

For medical practice, therefore, there appears to be an increased necessity to bear in mind the psychic aspect in any case of insomnia and its correction. Hypnotics which contain cortical sedatives will be more efficient, and all the more so because the sphere of affect is becoming damped down by them. Such an effect of damping down, in some cases, implies and even equals the partial relief of mental tension and the dissolution of affectively accentuated thought-elements, comparable with an analytical effect. This implies also the usefulness of administering sedatives (bromides, valerian) in the course of the afternoon. The pure hypnotics seem not to do full justice to the psychological aspect. It might be mentioned once more, that already in the first phase of a psychoanalytic treatment, incidental or additional insomnia frequently disappears. In spite of the well-known fact that the amount of remembered dream-material increases, on account of the necessity, pertaining to the method, of recollecting and reporting the dreams, the quality of sleep yet considerably improves ; because the analytical process, by reason of its specific character, unburdens the affect-mechanism. In every case where the conditions allow, longer analytical examination should play an eminent rôle in the treatment of functional sleep-disturbances ; and such functional insomnia ought to be supposed everywhere, where there is *no* reason to surmise a circulatory or other organic pathological brain-process. The fact that a satisfactory sexual experience facilitates sound sleep, is based similarly on its effect, diminishing the mental tension, and positively influencing the spheres of emotions. In every case, where there is noticeable a reverse influence on sleep, there surely a pathological state exists, based on certain complexes present, and an analysis, if only brief, is indicated.

The fact that indigestion and similar enteral disturbances might unfavourably affect sleep, has been always recognised and practically considered. Yet, even quite small dyskineses, subliminal for self-perception, of the abdominal organs, might initiate disturbances of sleeping and dreaming. This possibility follows logically from our expositions above, according to which organic stimulations are a constant source of dreaming and present a constant object of the affect-energetic processes. The present author once suggested, therefore, that in order to eliminate such minor tensions of the organs, sleeping drugs should contain also papaverin or its derivatives. However, so far no final and conclusive opinion could be gained as to the value of such a measure.

SUMMARY

The dream process has to be considered as a purposive, biological phenomenon, essential to normal life. It is included in the affect-regulative processes of the nervous system. Sleep disturbances originate mostly from dysfunctions of the affect-metabolism. The dream-image, remembered after awaking, appears to represent a kind of metabolic end-product of the dream-energetic process. Its diagnostic value in the treatment of psychogenic troubles is not only equal to the rôle assigned to material laboratory investigations, but surely exceeds it. That energetic quality which, as organic stimulation, influences dream formation, is similar, or even equal in kind, to that energetic material, which, ensuing from psychic experiential sources, represents an essential part of dream-formation. The aim of treatment of sleep disturbances should lie, in most of the cases, in a positive furthering, and relieving of, the affect-metabolism.

CHAPTER XI

ARCHAIC AND INFANTILE TRAITS

SOME authors (as Freud, H. Ellis, Jung, etc.) emphasise that dreams show many infantile traits, as well as traits corresponding to primitive levels of human evolution. One peculiarity of dream-formation, that of personifying processes occurring within the psychosomatic organism, does indeed reveal an obvious relation to both these aspects. It is true that the baby plays with parts of his own body, as if they were external objects, and also that the small child speaks of himself in the third person, i.e., without making any distinction—in his language at least—between " I " and " You ". There *is*, therefore, a certain similarity between the objectification, personification of subjective phenomena, as effectuated by the dream, and the behaviour of the child. I think, without however going very deeply into this problem, that any far-going conclusion is not quite cogent. The speaking of oneself in the third person (" John is a good boy to-day " instead of " I am a good boy to-day ") is certainly indicative of a yet incomplete ego-formation in the child ; but essentially it is a provisional adoption of how the adults of his surroundings are speaking about him and about others. It is difficult to know how much true objectification is implied in such a manner of speech, or in the playing of babies with their toes. I have pointed out (Ch. V) that the dream-ego certainly " knows " that all the dream-elements actually belong to *one* homogeneous, unitary personality, but it experiences *for other reasons* the " parts " of it in a personified and dramatised form. Similarly, the child employs modes of personification and dramatisation in his expressions (in play and speech), without having, however, a split self-perception in a true, deeper sense. It is obvious that his imagination *allows* such a playful objectification, without being inhibited by the sense for reality. Yet the phenomenon of externalising his bodily parts implies probably play rather than any deeper deficiency.

More serious significance for our problem is to be found in references to the " savage ", the man as yet unexperienced in natural science who animates, personifies and externalises, i.e., views as "foreign apparitions" *his own feelings,* just as does the dream-ego. I would like to remark : *If* men of the earliest cultural levels dreamed differently than we do, or not at all, then we may see in the present modes of dream-representation, and also in " infantile " fashions of thinking and expressing oneself, such archaic mechanisms (without admitting, however, that they signify, and are at present, no more than simple remnants and traces). But if man has always dreamt as we do, has always experienced physiological and psychic events in a pictorial and dramatised fashion, then I would reverse this argument and surmise : the scientifically unexperienced primitive man has made use of his unconscious dream-mechanisms, and carried them over into the thinking of his waking life. In virtue of an unconscious realisation of the modes at work in the psychic depths and dreaming, he carried out his waking thinking and explaining in a similar fashion. This statement will probably encounter opposition ; but it may perhaps stimulate a few readers to give some thought to the problem. . . . It is, of course, quite possible that I am wrong in this hypothesis. But even if we were really dealing with mere " archaic " mechanisms, I should definitely refuse a too simple explanation. It has been maintained in this work that the " scenic experiencing " in the dream is possibly a mechanism, built into the rest of the physiological processes, a mechanism which, to us as we are nowadays, constitutes a physiological necessity, though perhaps not absolutely essential to maintain life, yet desirable and useful from the viewpoint of complete somato-psychic health. The archaic mechanisms, then, would be put at the service of this *experiencing-function* in present-day man. Only those who do not regard the dream-experience as being at work constantly, but as an image, a hallucination constituting a reactive product to a disturbing stimulus, and as *merely* the effect of such a stimulation, only they can logically doubt the physiological significance and necessity of the sleep-dream-experience, and implicitly deny the systematic and purposive use of the " archaic " mechanisms. But we cannot help seeing a " biological function " in the whole process of dreaming, all its detailed characteristics included. This question has been discussed in Ch. X from the viewpoint of " affect-economy ". The statements and suggestions there, however, must be supplemented by taking into special consideration also the formed, scenic *dream-images*. The dream is a true experience, the dream-scene is experienced. That which is being experienced in it, are functions and processes of the *psychosomatic ego*. In principle, it is the same, whether there occur in the dream an experiential perception of inner organic events, or a perception of external stimuli in their effect on the ego, or of psychic processes proper ; all three groups of phenomenon are only constituents of the ego-totality. *There is only one kind of dreaming within the human organism.* In dreaming, the whole psychoaffective content (the physical, organic stimuli are included, viz., Ch. X) is being " elaborated ", and the *total ego experienced.* It is as if it were a specially organised, intensified ego-feeling, which latter constitutes also an important aspect of the personality of our waking being.[1] The various dream images are parts, traces of this self-experiencing process occurring in sleeping. There is some formal justification for separating these images from the total dreaming-experience, and for viewing them, as already suggested, as some kind of final metabolic product. It is, however, an end-product which originates from the psychoaffective sphere, thus pointing to the infinite spheres of " mind " and of " life ". The explanations on affect-metabolism and the corresponding nomenclature should, therefore, not be misinterpreted as expressing a one-sided, purely materialistic and mechanistic viewpoint.

Personification, scenic dramatisation, and symbolism proper are, as far as I can see, related processes. They certainly are *so* in the dream. Thus symbolism, too, is an " archaic " mechanism. It plays the leading rôle in the world of ideation when one thinks vaguely, emotionally, without distinct and clear conception. We have seen that in the art and poetry of modern man, and similarly in dreaming, symbolic substitute-formation and representation indicate an extension of the content, through more abundant connections with associations. Restriction of such associations forms the essence of cognising, defining and realistic thinking, which tends to circumscribe its object. If sleep and dreaming really constitute a renovation of the psychosomatic personality, a descent into the depths and " primitive sources " of life, then a return to " archaic " forms must be connected with this ; not only because the " primitive " is intrinsically the older, the " source " ; but also because it is, as already mentioned, more abundant, more capable of accepting and giving new, extended, deepening

[1] Cf. pp. 59, 231.

contents. I do not propose to go any further into this nebulous, " philosophising " discussion ; as in the previous chapters, I much prefer to remain clear, uncomplicated in presentation, though not too profound. On the probable archaic origin of the individual dream-symbols, cf. Ch. VI ; the reader is also referred to the work of O. Rank on " Psychoanalytic Contributions to Mythus-research ".

It is here that the deep and interesting views of Jung should be, at least briefly, described. In his opinion—and he has supported his statements by extensive studies of culture-history —the deepest *unconscious* of the individual has its share in the historical collective psyche. Just as the body bears traces of its phylogenetic past, so also does the brain-function. Hence the *unconscious* contains inherited " patterns ", and he calls these images, expressing complexes, *archetypes*. Animals and persons of different type represent deeply rooted potentialities, primitive human tendencies. The interpretation of such elements can be found, according to this author, in different concepts of the mythus of all ages and nations. *Horse*, for instance, is such a widely found archetype, representing in dream the instinctive, animal, subhuman side in general ; at the same time, the lower regions of the body, as the source from where these animal drives take their origin. It can stand for the unconscious mind, representing the animal, non-human psyche. It symbolises also dynamic power which carries one, and occasionally carries one away, disregarding limitations and difficulties.

The bull, the ass, the pomegranate, and similarly lightning and the dance, symbolise in mythology and folk-lore the power of fertility and of healing, i.e., the " creative mana ", the more obvious, direct representation of which is the phallus. Jung states that the racial origin of some individuals can be recognised by the archetypes prevailing in their dreams.

I should like to add that I firmly believe that certain dream-patterns of each individual are inherited motifs. If the dream-images contain representations of the " psychosoma "—and this is the view propounded here—then it is only logical that there must be such inherited dream-patterns. I had, and have frequently, the impression when trying to trace the origin of my own dreams that for some dream-elements no effort succeeds in producing associations, recollections which point to the historical past of the individual. We all experience sometimes in dreams places, forests, houses of a peculiar character, which certainly do not fit into anything we might have experienced during our individual life, in reality or in painting. Apart from this phenomenon, the close dependence on the organic structure of dream-formation is bound to result in certain inherited modes of dream-representation. This, however, does not mean necessarily the archetypes of Jung, but rather some individual and intrinsic characters, pertaining to the closer family-gene.

The infantile element in dreams can be described as follows. Apart from the basic " infantile dream-stimulus " postulated by Freud, it must be admitted that the manifest dream really contains allusions to periods of life, lying far in the individual past. Associations are even more liable to lead there. In addition, we must look upon the relative lack of inhibitions, the disregard of social barriers, as well as the lack of consideration for what is possible and expedient, as an *apparent return* to an immature, infantile stage. But according to what has been said above, this means only a *formal* placing into the class of infantilisms. The dream is an intensified "ego-experience"; hence it follows automatically that barriers arising from social and ethical considerations cannot have the same strength as they do in shaping the waking life and its thinking. As regards the lack of logic and deficient consideration of concrete facts and physical barriers, we must remember that we are here dealing with personified ego-representations ; that the subconscious and dream-ego " knows " about the psychological fact that the inner, and not the outer, world is being dreamt. Hence, there is actually no reason for taking into consideration, at any rate, barriers belonging to the outer world of our life. In this connection, therefore, it is preferable to speak of *forms of infantile thinking*, rather than of its *essential quality*. The dream-experience makes use of these infantile forms of thinking, because they are, under certain circumstances obtaining within the psyche, more suitable for the purposes of dreaming, and because, on the other hand, *there is no reason for not employing* such illogical, unreal forms. *That mode and that process* is being used by the dream which will enable, at any particular moment, the most abundant elaboration of the ego-experience. *For dreaming is essentially one special way of ego-experiencing* [1] *; the latter, however, seems to be—because of its constant occurrence—a psycho-physiological need, an indispensable life-condition.*

[1] Cf. Ch. XII, p. 234.

CHAPTER XII

PROBLEMS OF INTERPRETATION [1]

(1) IN this chapter we shall draw some conclusions from our discussions, emphasising whatever may be of use for special dream-interpretation, as required and practised in psychotherapy. From the very close connection of the various constituents of the dreams—we have in mind here especially the simultaneous and intermixed representation of organic and psychic processes—follows necessarily the postulate to look upon the dream image as an *overdetermined* [2] *formation*. Since in the dream organogenic and psychic material coalesce into a unity (and we maintain that for the *subconscious* both constitute essentially quite similar stimulus-material), [3] it is certain also that different psychic elements, though of the most varied origin, may meet in one and the same dream-image. Fundamentally, there is only *one* total consciousness, not single thoughts. Similarly, there is only one, admittedly complicated dream-world, not individual, separate dream-elements. *Like every experience, the dream-experience is a unity.* Thus it is certain that historical and functional elements are present in the dream *simultaneously*, and similarly we have to suppose, in principle at least, that elements of the past, serving as a life-basis, attitudes of the present, and plans for the future, co-exist in every dream. The phenomenon of *condensation*, the existence of which, in respect of the individual dream-elements, was discovered and proved by Freud, is so fundamentally a much more general dream quality. Associations to the manifest dream also show that its elements belong to levels which differ greatly in content and temporal origin. But this condensation of the dream-image, unlimited in principle, is merely a theoretical postulate. In actual practice we find that not every dream-image allows us to penetrate to the same degree into the whole conglomeration of relations which, in principle, are supposed to lie at the back of the dream. Nevertheless, there is absolute justification in any given case *in trying* to trace these various relations and aspects.

[1] Add Ch. I (14).   [2] Occasioned simultaneously by several sources.
[3] Ch. X.

(2) I shall add here a few paragraphs which I published in 1933 in the journal *Psychoanalytische Praxis* under the title " Symptom und determinierende Komplexe im Traumbild ".[1] The interpretation of the few dreams given there may appear somewhat schematic ; this was the consequence of my endeavour to restrict the discussions to the most important and relevant points ; yet definitely due also to the fact that I was considerably younger at that time. All this, I hope, does not invalidate the argument of the article.

The classical investigations of H. Silberer have shown clearly that the dream-image *does not* deal only with the " ideal content ", i.e., with the " subject of our thinking and feeling," but also with the " state and functions of the psyche ". His investigations started from the close relation existing between the hypnagogic (ante-sleep) hallucinations on the one hand, and the waking thoughts and bodily positions, immediately preceding them, on the other. His conclusions could then be transferred to dreams proper.

I shall attempt to give first a brief account of Silberer's main discoveries, illustrating them through a dream investigated by me. An intelligent, middle-aged business man one day realised that the struggle between radicalism and conservatism had not been fought to a conclusion in the deeper levels of his mind. Nevertheless, he refused to occupy himself any further with the problem, because it was of no importance whatsoever for him. He felt too old and inert to put his convictions, based on mere feeling, into the frame of a detailed philosophical system. The following night he dreamed :

> **72a.** It is a question of *two books* by the famous mathematician, Poincaré, which are supposed *to be brought nearer* to each other, but which all the same remain *at a constant distance*.

The mathematician, Poincaré, is also famous for his books in defence of religion. His *two books* in the dream, according to the dreamer, point to the radical, materialistic Weltanschauung (mathematical way of thinking) and to the conservative (religious) one. In that part of the dream in which the two books " are supposed to be brought nearer to each other, but remain at a constant distance ", the inert way of thinking of the dreamer referred to above, i.e., his *psychic attitude* to the whole problem, is brought out graphically.

[1] Symptom and Determinative Complexes in the Dream-image.

The dreamer added that the dream-experience was accompanied by painful feelings and lasted for some time ; the images re-emerged again and again after short pauses. He also thought that it had been very cold that night and that he had been constantly engaged in retrieving his blankets, which kept sliding off him. This recollection brought forth a supplement to the dream as related :

72b.   The books appeared to be icy-cold. . . .

There is no doubt that this " icy-cold " feeling in the dream owed its inception to the cold night, or rather to the sliding-off of the blankets ; thus the two books whose failure to come together had created such a painful impression, reflected at the same time the ever-repeated attempts to retrieve the blankets. (Hence the frequent re-emergence of the dream.)

The property of the dream in virtue of which the state of the psyche and also that of the body is represented pictorially in the dream image, was called by Silberer " autosymbolism ".

The equal participation of thoughts, affective and organic processes in the " stimulation " of dreams, points to the close connection of the dreaming with the total of the physiological reactions and life processes in general, and suggests that the dreaming might carry a biological significance, essential for normal life. (Cf. Ch. X, where this aspect of the problem is discussed in detail.) A scientific theory which sees in the dream nothing but the deposit of subconscious events and of repressions, does not do justice to such a complicated and constant life phenomenon. I should not hesitate to ascribe to the dream-process a range of function, as extensive and important within the total sphere of physiological events as that of the circulation of the blood, of the alimentary, of the excretory or of the endocrine systems. While, however, all these organic systems represent relatively independent functional units, besides their ultimate action on the whole organism, the dream-process seems to collect stimuli, taking their origin from all the various fields, including, of course, the cerebro-psychic mechanism, in order to submit them to its regulative " working-up " process.[1] (In the customary way

---

[1] The fact that in the dream-image—i.e., the conscious product of the dream-producing process—the " psychic " influences are especially noticeable, is due in the first place to the greater difficulty of recognising the influence of somatic stimuli. The dreamer is able to give information about only a few subjectively felt organic processes. Furthermore, it is probable that the psychic events are

"organic" and "psychic" dream sources have been distinguished.) This view on the nature of the dream process may facilitate the understanding of some peculiarities of the dream-image; in particular that of the analytically discovered, but actually not yet explained, "*condensation*".[1] If the dream-process has the physiological task of regulating and elaborating (in a way, the true nature of which is not yet disclosed to us), all the stimulus-quanta, split off from the whole psychosoma, then the dream-image which originates from this activity must, of course, reflect all the energy-transformations taking place within the organism (as in the different organ-functions or with the conative and emotional processes, etc.). In this way a condensation of a doubled character originates : on the one hand somatogenic and psychogenic influences are being fused together, and on the other hand various different thought-elements are being compressed. The dream cited above clearly exemplifies this.

In a similar way we can explain the overt, symbolic or only half-suggested representation of parapathic [2] symptoms in the dream. There is an energetically charged complex in the subconscious psyche, pertaining and corresponding to the symptom, whether it be a pure psychic or an organ-neurotic one, even in those intervals when the patient is free from an attack. The excitation, impinging on the current dream-formation from this source, must inevitably affect also the dream-representation of this symptom. Thus, a neurotic asthmatic patient dreams now about a breath-taking duel, now about some large event where the window is violently opened, now about some over-crowded meeting, where he is hemmed in on all sides. In all these images there is some feature, suggesting the actions of the respiratory apparatus in the state of dyspnoea. The "breath-taking" duel contains the element of subjectively felt lack of breath ; the large crowd at the

actually more extensive than the "material-organic" processes. Cf. J. H. Schultz's statement in his *Lehrbuch der Psychotherapie* : "The body is only part of the Psyche".

[1] Cf. Ch. V, p. 127.

[2] An expression of Stekel, equivalent to the term "neurotic". Parapathy signifies "emotional disturbance, creating symptoms". Yet, primarily organic symptoms are also hinted at in the dream-image. In all organ-symptomatic cases the dream-element might originate from the subliminally always present symptom, and not necessarily from the underlying energetic complex. *We think, however, that even in "pure" organic cases it is the secondary or simultaneously present psychic content, grafted upon the pathological process, which brings about the influence on the psyche and on the dreaming.*

meeting, mirrors the bronchial spasm, as it hampers his breathing ; the violent opening of the window corresponds in its dynamism to his frantic efforts to end this spasm.

Those parts of the dream-image which contain an *autosymbolic representation of the patient's symptoms* offer us in their constituents highly valuable hints with regard to important complexes. I shall give three examples :

(i) This was the dream of a young man who was treated for erective difficulties :

> **73.** A station—there is great disorder. Several trains are ready to depart, but none of them move. There seems to have been a collision. . . . On one side one can see a heap of wreckage, and something longish and round projects from it. This object becomes longer and longer, one can see gradually more of it, till finally it turns out to be a *female's* leg.

This dream was accompanied by an *erection*. It is not difficult to recognise in the longish object which erects more and more, *the autosymbolic representation of the process of genital erection.* The female body belonging to the projecting leg, which is buried under the wreckage, points clearly to a *sadistic complex.* Indeed, there could be found in the patient's anamnesis a period of his youth, during which his sexual thinking was accompanied by markedly *masochistic* phantasies of " being beaten ".[1] (The object projecting more and more from the heap of ruins, signifies, at the same time, the process of analysis, in its striving for growing clearness.)

(ii) The following two dreams, both occurring during one night, were reported by a young man who was suffering from the feeling, that " there were no normal relations between him and the world around him ". Everything seemed strange and he felt himself similarly strange to others.

> **74.** This dream takes place in Spain, at the time of the Inquisition. I am sitting with some people who have, on their heads, very high, pointed hats. There is somebody underneath the table (male or female), who attempts fellatio on me. Suddenly the myrmidons of the Inquisition come in and we have to flee. . . .

Association : Memory of a one-day relation with a man who

---

[1] Conscious masochism is based on primary, repressed sadism. In fact, both tendencies are in several cases simultaneously present.

carried out fellatio on him ; this experience ended for my patient in dissatisfaction and disappointment.

> **75.** I am going through the streets of Paris in an excursion bus ; for hours we see nothing but endless tramlines. I am very disappointed.

In the first dream the dreamer finds himself in a *strange country* ; the time of the action is also very remote (400 years ago). This is a picturalisation of the subjectively felt abyss between the patient and the world in general, i.e., *an illusion to the symptom which is being treated*. (At the same time there is an indication of analytical resistance ; the complex should remain *foreign* to consciousness.) In the second dream this feeling is represented by the *endless*, and apparently aimless, drive through the streets of Paris, where one expects so many enjoyable sights. (Here also we find an expression of analytical resistance : a determination not to get anywhere, to maintain the status quo.) The first dream contains the homosexual *fellatio complex* (see also the pointed hats) which is alluded to in the second dream by the Parisian pleasure trip (" french love "). At the same time these two dreams illustrate an observation which I have described elsewhere,[1] viz., that often the dreams of the same night contain in their manifest form or in the associations given to them, the same motifs, and that these identities point to important complexes. (Cf. also the repeated theme of *disappointment*.) Up to the time of his treatment the patient expected too much from his fellow humans, i.e., bodily tenderness ; consequently, he was *disappointed* and dissatisfied by the usual relations which were, of course, much less close than he demanded. Hence his morbid feeling of remoteness from the world.

(iii) A girl suffering from an extrapyramidal tremor, greatly increased by a psychic conflict,[2] dreamed several times :

> **76.** I am driving in a *black car, which shakes* so much that I almost fall out.

The association given to the car was *hearse*. The patient's basic complex was rooted in violent feelings of hatred and jealousy towards her sisters, whom she considered more success-

---

[1] " The Different Dreams of the Same Night." (Cf. also Ch. IV (7).)
[2] The recent psychic trauma occurred during her febrile illness, after which the slight " postencephalitic " symptoms appeared. First hypnotherapy, and later analytical " katharsis " brought about a considerable relief for a long time.

ful in social life. *The shaking of the car alludes to the tremor, the black car to the* (openly admitted) *hatred and death-wishes.* (There is also an allusion to the analytic " shaking up ", which makes repressed contents " fall out ".)

These examples show how the dream-representation of the symptom on the one hand, and certain actions and events in the dream on the other hand, are built up, so to speak, on the same " dynamic frame " ; the supplementary and embellishing elements which are added to this foundation point to important complexes, influential for the life of the dreamer. I once formulated this briefly : *The dream-picture of the symptom is painted with the lines and colours of the complexes.*[1] The fact that an allusion to the *analytic situation* is usually woven into the dream is explained by the fact of transference, i.e., the sub-conscious tendency to transfer all affectively coloured psychic tendencies, including those ensuing from the individual com-plexes (pathological and normal sentiments) to the analyst and his work. Thus the state of the analysis at any time is also represented by means of the complex—and symptom-colours. (Cf. Ch. IX.)

This rule of interpretation can, of course, be applied to any kind of dream-material. As examples I may at random quote two dreams cited by other writers. One of the several dreams of an ereutophobic (blushing) patient, which all confirm the " condensation rule " outlined above (as far as the necessary associations are added), runs : [2]

> 77. I accuse my fiancée, take my flash-light and bang it on the floor till the glass breaks.

The blushing is suggested by the flashing of the light. Throwing away the lamp relates to the death-wish against the suspected fiancée (extinction of light or life) ; and also to the analytical resistance. All this is contained in a *single situation-image.*

Another simple and instructive dream is the following.[3] The young man who dreamed it was suffering from examin-ation-fear :

> 78. I am standing before the examination-committee clad only in my shirt. I feel very embarrassed.

---

[1] *V. Kongressber. für Psychotherapie,* 1930. (Report on the V. Congress for Psychotherapy.)
[2] Kratter in *Psych. Praxis,* Vol. 2, No. 4.   [3] Feldman *ibid.*

Here also we find the symptom, complex (exhibitionism) and the analytical situation united into one dream-situation.[1] (3) The multiformity of symbolic substitution is almost unlimited. States of the body and of the psyche, instinctive drives and different mental tendencies, are all represented in most varied ways and forms. *Organic stimuli, instinctive tendencies and attitudes may be represented in dreams by persons, animals, objects or even places of a certain significance.* This fact justifies us in considering all possible substitute formations, when looking for the meaning and context of the dream. One and the same image may portray a relationship to the outer world, to persons or events, and indicate at the same time a functional content, i.e., a state of the psyche. When in dream No. 12 the full basin represents the full bladder, at the same time it stands for the motif of the difficulty in which the disturbed sleeper finds himself. The rôle taken here by the full and disturbing bladder, in other cases may be played by a different objective event in the outer world or by a real person. We find in every dream-image which pictorialises the reaction to a disturbing stimulus or to an external condition, the representation of *that* stimulating factor, and at the same time the representation of the ensuing and accompanying psychic state. Frequently it is the same dream-fragment which portrays both, as in the example just quoted. Yet, since the dream contains in fact far more than simply the reaction to some particular event or stimulus, which we have come incidentally to know, we may always try to interpret the same image or dream-fragment in various ways, even though there is no apparent connection between one motif and the others. If we were in the position to grasp at any moment all those elements, which in their totality make up the actual state of the psyche, or its cross-section at any given moment, then we should also be in the position to see all the connections. But as this is not possible, we may, for practical purposes, grope in various directions from the original dream-element, suspecting various attitudes and facts behind this element, even though the intrinsic connections of all these individual items and complexes are hidden from us.

Let us consider first a simple example which illustrates this. The following dream was reported by a doctor, an autistic man, who was *suffering from general difficulties of adjustment* :

[1] Dream-situation is one simultaneous part of the more or less complicated dream-event, one individual " situation " of the whole story.

79. There is a funny red-cheeked man in front of me : I undertake an anal exploration. We joke together ; he smiles cynically.

From the associations we learn that his father had red cheeks, and also used to smile cynically. Furthermore, the face reminded the patient of a colleague who annoyed him by his constant criticism and his conceit. Finally, he admitted that he had been suffering from pruritus ani and was wont to scratch himself so badly, even during sleep, that his pyjamas became full of holes.

It is more than probable that we are dealing here with an organically stimulated dream. It seems obvious that the man had undertaken an "anal exploration" on himself during sleep. Added to this is his "objective" interpretation in reference to his father ; the latter often hurt him by his ceaseless and unjust criticism, and kept him altogether too much under paternal control. At the end of the therapeutic session we succeeded also in discovering in the dream his mockery of the analyst and his derision of the analytical treatment as mere superficial conversation. This was indicated jocosely by the patient in his behaviour and his remarks, which both should be regarded as complementary associations to the dreams previously related. ("You are not very tired, my daily work is different", and so on.) In this example there is no apparent association between the organic stimulus and the various psychic motifs. One might, perhaps, assume that the pruritus ani was itself of psychic origin, or at least intensified by some complex ; perhaps even directly connected with the patient's attitude towards his father ; or that the patient puts himself in the place of his analyst, and, in turn, wants to examine him from homosexual tendencies ? However, these suppositions could hardly be regarded as self-evident, as there was not anything to confirm them.

The connection appears clearer in the following example. A young female patient, who was suffering from agoraphobia and precordial pressure (the latter was the consequence of a slight hyperthyroidism), dreamed :

80. I see a dish with a mouse inside. The mouse is to die. Then it is a woman who is to die. I wake up with heart-pressure ; I have the feeling I might die.

The associations lead in various directions ; but one thread running through them all is clearly recognisable. First came the thought of her *mother* who was suffering from *heart-pains*. Then she thought of a man, the lover of her mother, who spoke about a mouse when she met him last. She felt hurt by the intimacy between the two, and was ashamed on that account. She cannot eat ; everything disgusts her, as a mouse in a dish does. Her own " friend " (she is also unhappily married), has a name similar to that of her mother's friend. Her conscience troubles her because of her own love affair, and she feels she ought not to bear a grudge against her mother because of hers. Her husband speaks derisively about the mother's love-affair. She then remembers an obscene story her father once told about a mouse. Her father is jealous of his wife ; but he tolerates the existing conditions. He drinks, and for years he has slept apart from her mother.

We need not add any further explanation. The coherent condensation of the different details behind the dream-image is obvious. Let us remember that the manner of producing associations differs from one patient to the other ; and even the same person associates differently on different occasions. In many cases intermediate links remain unconscious ; also the distance of the association from the initial dream element varies considerably (Ch. IV (6)). Discoveries which apply, say, to ten per cent of all dreams, may be generalised quite justifiably. It follows from the intrinsic nature of dream formation that an exact investigation of the material meets with enormous difficulties.

(4) Just as the subconscious part of a psychic content is not completely congruent with its conscious counterpart (cf. pp. 63–6), just as repressed elements become also different from their original content, similarly we find that the dream is not simply a condensed, abbreviated formation, which is essentially identical with the total of its " latent " content. I should say that the dream and its parts *correspond* to a multitude of original elements, like two things which belong to each other, yet which are not identical and even not necessarily similar. *Dream-interpretation, then, is essentially a conclusion* a posteriori. We cannot say definitely that the various elements and relations which we find in the associations, are really contained in the dream image, *really* make up the " content " of the dream. But there is a degree of probability that they indicate the sources, i.e., the external experiences, or self-perceptions, which have supplied the deep-consciousness with that material,

the derivatives of which are woven into the dream.   But apart from this genetic point of view, we have to consider the dream image as a whole, possessing *one* unitary, self-sufficient content, to delimit which may, however, be frequently difficult.   In the tree likewise, we know *that there is a root*, but its ramifications are too extensive to allow its exposure as an unmutilated whole. Theoretically, however, we *can* delimit the dream content proper.   *The dream creates a new situation from its constituent elements ; everything that pertains to the delineation of this situation* (though the dreamer does not describe explicitly all the details of the implicit content), *is definitely part of the dream.*   As pointed out elsewhere, the intuitive interpreter should feel himself into the dream-event (" empathy "), should let the image in its totality pass through his own psyche, let it enter his mental eye ;   then his own inner fund of experience will supply him with the necessary supplements ;   with whatever is needed to transform the verbalised dream-image into a " living content ". Just in the same manner as *the apparently monochromatic ray of sunlight is de-composed into its individual and differently coloured components, by being passed through a prism.*[1]   Every image which belongs to the dream, every object which plays a part in the delineation of a scene, signifies *something*, means " intrapsychic life ".[2]   But, again, this is only theory.   In actual practice we have to rest content with discovering single motives, and for psychotherapeutic purposes actually only certain elements and relations are important.   *The primary significance of the manifest dream* is, of course, a natural presupposition.   If the dream-mechanism finds it necessary to create the manifest dream, then it is not justifiable to take it as entirely non-essential.

A neurotic asthmatic patient wakes up with badly impeded breathing and remembers this dream :

81.   I had to *fight with a lion in a small room* ;   I was terribly afraid and threw the window open in order to escape.

When one puts oneself into this situation and pictures to oneself the narrow room, the threatening beast of prey so near, the tension, the fear, the sudden stopping of the breath in frightened expectation, the thoughts and alternating plans of escape ;   and at the same time the occasional, momentary admiration for the mighty king of beasts, the feeling of one's own smallness, of succumbing . . .   (I am only describing

---

[1] *Intuitive Dream-Interpretation*, 1930.   .   [2] Cf. p. 26.

the most superficial and obvious reactions)—then we have not only *a plastic representation of breathing difficulties*, of bronchial spasm and of the fight for dilation of the bronchi (throwing open the windows), but also some idea of the fullness of feelings in such a serious state of danger to one's life.

I add that in this case we are dealing with an incompetent yet conceited psychopath, who knew only *one* ethical law— that of the altruism of others towards him ; a man who reck- lessly bowed and scraped before the successful and the influ- ential, while at the same time he cunningly plotted behind their backs. In considering this, I think, there is some justifi- cation for interpreting the narrow room also [1] as a represent- ation of his *narrow horizon* and of his *limited, encumbered mental flexibility*, and the lion as a representation of those he superficially admired, but, deep down, hated because of their success and power. At the same time, the *lion* alludes to the writer, against whose analytical efforts he was prepared to fight (Löwe = lion in German).

I once had to treat a difficult neurotic because of his anxiety states. One of his early dreams was :

> **82.** I see a working-man handling a saw-like instrument. He seems to move it up and down, in that rural manner of cutting straw for cattle. I think *I am* the one who is doing the cutting ; also the one who is being cut.

I do not remember the exact wording of the dream, nor the associations ; the material is not now available. But I remember vividly that I expressed to Dr. Stekel (on whose instruction I treated the patient in Vienna), my purely intuitive suggestion, and judging only from the first plastic impression of the dream, that somehow we were dealing with the problem of masturbation and sadistic tendencies. The instrument and its rhythmic movements suggested to me the rhythm of sexual excitement, especially as there was in the dream a feeling that the dreamer was the individual doing the work, and at the same time the object which is being worked upon. Only after three months was I able to prove that the patient was under the sway of a *sadistic rape-phantasy*, which constituted the accompanying background of his masturbation in his early youth, and which was still being experienced by him, though

---

[1] It was noted that the greatest number of dream-events takes place in a com- paratively small space. Cf. Ch. II, p. 52, where a general explanation (not incompatible with the present one) was given.

quite subconsciously, during his auto-erotic acts as an adult. The evil consequences of this phantasy, i.e., his illness, is indicated by the fact that he is being " cut ". But in the same image (he cuts and is being cut) the fact of his compulsory auto-eroticism too finds expression. If one looked at this dream-image too objectively, too much " from a distance ", one could hardly find anything meaningful in it, least of all the suspected and subsequently confirmed facts. It cannot be emphasised too strongly that the interpreter should look upon the dream-text as the image of *a situation*, and put himself into it. (Cf. also Ch. II, p. 31.)

(5) It is a commonly accepted view in modern dream-interpretation that present difficulties in one's life, cause in dreams the re-appearance of older life-situations, or even of remote infantile memories, the contents of which show some kind of similarity and relation to the present. Purely technic-ally, we are dealing here with an associative connection and awakening. Dynamically, this phenomenon should be inter-preted as revealing the *continuity of psychic life through all its various periods and stages*. It is only natural that one's orient-ation in the present reflects one's previous experiences, and tries to gain advice and inspiration from a re-living of the past. This is, however, intelligible when the revived memories deal with the successful overcoming of difficulties ; when they give solace and inspiration in a difficult present. Even more intelligible is this connecting mechanism, when purely agree-able and beautiful memories are produced and re-lived. One understands the purpose and usefulness of awakening similar associations in the subconscious, by a happy situation in the present, in order to strengthen the depth of the emotional experience of the moment. The representation in the dream is, of course, no more than a visible trace, a symbol, of the actual, full subconscious processes.

A young man, very much in love, dreams :

83. I go to see my girl-friend in Australia, but only get near the town where she lives. There I see an old couple.

The dreamer was afraid that a difference of ten years in age might have bad consequences in the proposed marriage. But the aged couple in the dream reminded him of a similar case. There, too, the same age-difference had been present, and yet they had lived harmoniously 'till death parted them.

But what useful purpose can the connecting recollection of a disagreeable event of the past have for the psyche of the dreamer ? What is the possible advantage of dreaming about the mishaps of the past, when the present is creating difficulties enough ? Analysis in such cases will usually succeed in discovering the deeper content, and the more far-reaching connections, which go beyond the simple recollection of such unfortunate events. But, in general, we may point out that the traumatogenic shock-capacity of an actual event is lessened, the more prepared the psyche is, the more counter-forces, comparable to "anti-bodies" it has developed and stored in the past. We know, of course, that the reverse might also be true. An infantile trauma can pave the way for the pathogenicity of later events, which by themselves would not be intense enough, and which succeed in overthrowing the balance of the person only because they can proceed along paths, already constructed and facilitated. This, however, does not alter the fact, that counter-forces, psychic antibodies, are also present. And so in such cases, the dream's function of connecting up with the unpleasant past, signifies that the antibodies needed by the present situation *have* been mobilised. Essentially, therefore, the function of such disagreeable dreams is similar to that of happy dream-memories, i.e., *the positive furthering of the psyche.*[1]

From the point of view of affect-economy, the process discussed might be described in the following way. Any emotional state strives towards conceptual shaping, towards "understanding self-perception". An elation or depression, at first only felt, connects with an appropriate content. This seems to be a human biological need. An "understood" elation is deeper, and similarly, a "conceived" depression or anxiety is more bearable. There seems to be in any emotional situation an *excess of affect*, not quite covered by conscious conceptual content. *The dream-world of the night makes up for this lack, and in presenting deposits of past experiences and shaping them into new combinations*, achieves in such a way a filling in with formed conceptual mental content, of the surplus affect-material.[2]

(6) I have borrowed the expression *connection* (Anknüpfung)

---

[1] Cf. Ch. I, pp. 4 5.
[2] This process is, therefore, not a mere "rationalisation and motivation" of the emotional condition but a purposive, useful event. As is well known, older dream-theories regarded dreams as an "attempt at giving reasons" for sensations during sleep.

from Bjerre (Stockholm).   It seems to me to say more than the kindred idea " regression ", because it implies an active, purposive aim ;   whereas the process of regression means frequently a passive, weak " retreat " to former positions.   The author mentioned has treated in the most clear way the present problem.   I found a certain intrinsic similarity, though not in the individual material and not in the special way of present-ation, between his basic dream-conception and mine.   His book, however, came to my notice, through the kindness of the author, only at a time (at the end of 1938) when the general outline and foundation of my work could not be changed considerably.   I propose in my Special Dream-Interpretation to consider his point of view as far as critical investigation and my own experience might find this expedient.[1]

He does *not* reach the conclusion, as I do, with regard to the purely disagreeable dream-recollections, but one of his examples is, in fact, a very good illustration of my hypothesis. A young patient, suffering from agoraphobia and other anxiety symptoms, dreamed :

> **84.**   I am going to the w.c. on the ground-floor of our house, where we used to live, when I was a child.   My mother runs to tell me that someone is coming ;   she then goes to the door to prevent this somebody coming in.

" The patient's father was a drunkard.   Panic broke out among the children when they saw him coming home at night. Everyone sought refuge where he could.   The patient remem-bers how, when he was very small, he crept under the table, or hid in a corner.   The mother was the acme of kindness and love, and tried to protect the children in every way possible. However, there is little wonder that the patient encountered considerable difficulties in escaping entirely from his terror, a terror which childhood had branded into his soul and which formed a foundation-stone in his character.   In the dream he conjures up the memory of the good, protecting power of his past life."

Being ignorant of this patient's detailed case history I should not add anything to the author's discussion ;   but the reasons given for the anxiety states, and the interpretation of the dream, do not seem to me to be appropriate to such serious

[1] Bjerre's book describes his individual, special way of interpretation, in an attractive, poetic fashion ;   it does not deal with the basic problems discussed in this work.

symptoms, from which the patient was suffering in his adult life. As far as the interpretation goes, it is without doubt correct. The dream deals in fact with the anxiety, and also with the possible defence. What I have called " unconscious immunisation through the development of mental antibodies ", is *personified* in this dream. It is the mother, who in the dream keeps the intruder out ; yet this intruder signifies essentially the illness, the pathogenic complexes ; and accordingly the mother-person symbolises the inner protective forces. She signifies the power which can " tie down ", or nullify the anxiety. Again, there is little doubt that the person who is prevented from coming in, is the patient himself ; *he* suffers from agoraphobia, from inhibition in moving about and going out ; also, there is a definite *reason* which prevents him from walking freely. Perhaps the fear of going out in the evenings, as his father used to do ? The fear of so causing pain to the mother ? Thus desecrating her memory after she died ?

(7) Bjerre says, " Even the most superficial observation shows that during sleep there is an actualisation of events, of which we have not thought for many years, and which we believed we had long forgotten. Closer investigation shows that dream-images are often reproductions of earlier events, which we cannot under any circumstances recall to memory. A male patient dreamed he was a small boy playing with a little girl. The girl upset what he was building and made it collapse. He was furious and bit the girl in the arm. He could not remember at all ever having taken part in such a scene, but his mother remembered the scene and confirmed that it agreed in every detail with the dream. Experiences like this which are quite obvious, as well as others with which we become acquainted only through the analysis of the sub-conscious, point to the fact that the subconscious has a special connecting function. By means of the dream-formation, details of the past are continually re-introduced into conscious-ness, are thus prevented from sinking into such depths that they cannot be recovered. Those of our experiences which are not at the moment accessible to consciousness are thus kept in touch with consciousness, so that in case of necessity associ-ation with them may become easier.

" This connecting function of the dream-formation is rein-forced considerably by formation of symbols. When this function takes a hand and condenses masses of experiences, perhaps a whole period of the dreamer's life, into one single image, then all the material which is contained in this synthesis, is re-connected with consciousness. Dream-formation thus causes not only a connection of single details, but also of whole ' conglomerations ' of past experience. But this is not all. Through the *constancy and continuity existing in the process of dreaming*, there is created a connection with this dream-continuity, which fact greatly contributes to the preservation of the cohesion and the unity of mental life as a whole.   When things are going against the grain and we despair, then we revert to the life-sources of the past—intentionally or instinctively—or perhaps usually both together.   It seems likely that the dream with its strong synthetic tendency, will attempt to tap simultaneously several life-sources of the past, and make them coalesce into *one stream*."

" A young mother with two children once dreamed the following dream :

> **85.**   I saw two beautiful white calves in a landscape ;   then I saw the cow, their mother.

" The patient identified the landscape at once with a place which played an important rôle in her very happy childhood. This was the most beautiful place she had seen until then—a perfect paradise.   The calves of the dream-experience could be derived from a scene she had seen in the Norwegian mountains, where, the summer before, she had passed a month, happy in every respect.   When she came home and showed photographs of them to the children they became wild with excitement and demanded to have the animals at all costs.

" The dream connects up with the happiness of her childhood, with the wandering in the mountains and with her motherhood, and attempts to bring strength to the patient from all these sources."

These interpretations of Bjerre may sound poetical and, therefore, " unscientific ".   Thoughts and feelings expressed in them are, however, true to life, are possible contents of human minds, and consequently of the subconscious, and thus not far from the world of dreams.

Bjerre points rightly to the importance of the feeling of psychic continuity, without going into the question at any length.   Yet the meaning of this idea will be clear to every psychologist.   The psyche is orientated towards *unity*, towards constancy. Sudden, surprising events would exert a devastating influence, unless they could be fitted into this mental unity. As organic food has to be transformed and assimilated into the human and individual kind of organ-albumen, so psychic events must be fitted into the totality of the unified ego. *Connection* is one important step towards this mental assimilation in the opinion of this author.

(8) *Stereotyped dream-motifs and their interpretation.* The appearance of stereotyped dream-images, i.e., dreams which recur in the life of an individual in the same or similar form, had been frequently discussed in its psychoanalytical significance. Quite logically they were interpreted by the authors as the expression of certain complexes, which are significant for the basic mental structure of the dreamer. From the formal point of view they are mostly short and of a simple structure. I may remind the reader here of the dreams which reflect the influence of strong organic stimuli and which also show this formal property. It is as if such stereotyped dreams had become " organic " parts of the individual. Single recurring motifs in the dreams must be viewed in the same way. I know an individual who often dreams of mice ; another of my patients dreamed frequently about a cat and a dog ; a third always introduced into his erotic dreams the following motif : he causes pain to his partner during coitus, and then consoles her. This last patient suffered from erectional impotence since his marriage ; he could not achieve defloration till two years after the first attempt, and seems to re-live this theme in the dream-motif mentioned. He experiences complete satisfaction in these dream-events. It might be noted that after three months' treatment he felt cured to such an extent that for the first time in 15 years he was able to have intercourse with his wife three to four times a week.[1] The success was due purely to the—surely inadequate—treatment, and not to any change in his private life-conditions. Unfortunately, the analysis could not be continued and I do not know whether the type of his dreams changed in a considerable degree.

One of the patients mentioned above suffered from masochistic phantasies ; he masturbated while he imagined being forced into intercourse by a strong, hefty female. The analysis

---

[1] One has, of course, not frequently the opportunity to achieve such quick success in chronic, neglected cases.

made it probable that his repeated dreams about a cat and a dog who were always fighting, had some bearing upon his sado-masochism.

In the first example mentioned a sister complex seemed to be hidden behind the mouse motif. In one of his dreams the mouse actually was changed into the sister. I cannot go into the analytical description of these cases in this book. I propose rather to add some considerations about the nature of this phenomenon. If there is anything which can make the *constancy of unconscious psychic life* clear and obvious to us, it is the recurrent stereotyped dream. If there is anything which can illustrate the remaining actuality of past events, the continued subconscious " life " of impressions and complexes, it also is these dreams. In addition, they contribute to our knowledge of the nature of symbolism ; or rather, they enable a deeper insight into the relation between content and representation.

Let us consider the case of the man who dreamed about mice. It is hardly necessary to stress that neither mice as a species, nor a particular mouse, would be likely to play a formative rôle in his inner life. Even though it was possible, during a long analysis, to show, or at least to make probable, *why* the mouse had been chosen as the bearer of a certain psychic constellation, yet there is, in fact, no deep, no essential, connection. It does not suffice to answer that the mouse is a well-known sexual symbol. This symbolic equation does not seem clearly founded in conscious thinking. Under no condition does the idea of the mouse, running into its hole, lie in the direction of conscious, normal sexual " feeling ". *By this we mean to say that in principle the symbolical substitution in dream, is not restricted to what is consciously intelligible and fully explicable.* Other different, unconscious mechanisms are at work, into whose functioning we shall never gain full insight. *Yet from this fact we may conclude that a too scrupulous exactitude in interpretation is unjustified as long as we are cautiously groping among conjectures.* The intuitive dream interpreter ought to have, and to employ, a vivid imagination, but should not publish every occasional idea and finding as a definitive result of a far-reaching validity. It is possible that for a particular patient, at a certain stage of his life or of the treatment, *one* dream-object may carry a certain significance ; then never again. The particular interaction of inner forces, as present in his subconscious at that time, may never recur. We see the reverse phenomenon in the recurring dream motifs. Here a symbolical equation becomes fixed, securely implanted, in that particular patient's psyche ; this is a certain confirmation of the constancy of symbolism, as posited by Freud for the sexual field ; yet it is so, only from the individual point of view. It really appears as if we have in such cases a constant relation (constant for that individual) between symbol-representation and content. We may also point to the parallel case of psychogenic symptoms. There also a fixed overt expression stands for a pathological mental constellation, i.e., there is a subjective and constant symbol for a complex. (Allers actually has compared the symptom to the symbol, regarding it as a kind of overt symbolic expression.)

(9) Analytical experience and theoretical considerations, however, will give us an even deeper insight. It is true that we can make the symptom disappear through an interpretive solution. Yet why does this process take so long ? Whence the necessity to treat the whole personality at the same time, and not only to consider the symptom ? It is so, because the individual symptom is, in fact, rich in content ; it is fed not only by *one* mental complex, but by a whole series of complexes, though they all might flow into *one* terminal stream. The "main complex" is responsible for the *form*[1] of the symptom, and, at times too, for the nucleus of the neurosis. Sometimes, however, the symptom is rather the overt expression of the *last*, actual event, which made the illness manifest. But in no case of chronic psychic illness is there only one root to the symptom. There are similar conditions for the stereotyped dreams and recurrent dream-motifs. The number of contents which are expressed by them, is all the larger the more experiences have become grafted upon the original one in the course of time. As time goes on, it may happen that the grafted content becomes superior to the original content with regard to extent or present significance. One must remain flexible in the interpretation of such rigid symbols and stereotyped dreams, if one does not gain the impression, through therapeutic success, of having already come to the root of the matter.

I shall explain this thesis in connection with obsessional neuroses. Stekel had noticed that patients suffering from obsessional ideas and compulsions (Zwangsparapathie), could

---

[1] Compare the " pathogenetic " and " pathoplastic " factors in the case of symptoms.

be helped along to a more rapid recovery at a certain stage of treatment, if one could " tear away " from them the " secret ", round which, like a nucleus, the illness was built. As I see it after a study of various cases, this " secret ", i.e., the traumatic experience, has left sometimes a noticeable trace in the symptomatology ; it is not always possible, however, to find this close connection between symptom and the ultimate secret. I remind the reader of a case which I have described briefly already in Ch. IV, pp. 106–7. It is the young man who was afraid of dying, if he should marry. There were a number of different complexes of considerable importance, all of which caused him, even consciously, much trouble and remorse. In the course of treatment, and during the progressive unravelling of all these complexes, considerable relief was experienced. Yet he did not get rid entirely of his compulsion and complaints. Five months of treatment had already passed and this made me decide to attempt a direct attack. He told me once the following dream :

> **86.** I am rowing in a boat with my late brother ; it is dark. Suddenly the moon rises.

Thereupon I said, with a resoluteness and certainty which in fact I did not feel, " You are consciously keeping something important from me. I surmise you have played sexually with your brother." (I was taking, of course, a considerable risk by doing this.) At first the patient tried to deny my supposition ; but as I was becoming convinced of the correctness of the " accusation ", I gave him a sound dressing down, telling him that he was insincere, did not want to get better, etc. Then followed a full confession : he had once slept with his brother and had had intercourse with him. As far as I can account for my intuitive interpretation, it followed presumably the following train of thought : The moon, suddenly rising, reminded me of a " sudden erection " ; rowing in the boat together in the dark night suggested to me the " sleeping and playing with each other ". I also remembered an earlier dream of this patient, in which he had seen this brother in girl's clothes. If one brings all these single elements together, my assumption will appear, at least partly, supported. It would perhaps not be quite convincing for everybody. But I had the feeling of being right. I have shown elsewhere [1]

---

[1] " *Confirmation of Intuitive Interpretation,*" 1934.

how, in the course of analysis, the reflected image of the structure of the illness builds itself up gradually in the subconscious of the analyst, from the various single elements, impressions he receives from the patient ; this is comparable with a *photographic negative*. This appears to be the source of his intuition, and also the ground of the so-called countertransference (emotional attitude of the therapist toward his patient). At all events, the obsession disappeared after one more week. This example shows that *there is*, as suggested by Stekel, such a nucleus in obsessional neurosis. I should like to add, however, that this " nucleus-secret " is *not* contained in our case in the obsessive-idea. It is, at the best, hinted at from afar ; through the motif of dying—the brother had died some time after the sexual event mentioned. It was obvious from the whole material, however, that the mother—and father—conflict was at least as important for causing his break-down, and for influencing the deeper structure of the neurosis. The mother-conflict was closer in content to the obsessive idea ; she had urged him *not* to marry a certain girl, except *over her dead body*.

(10) The case is similar with the stereotyped dream-motifs. They contain, on the one hand, as a core, the deposits and traces of a certain experience, or a certain complex ; but on the other hand the affective, latent content which lies at the back of them is surely made up of more and of diverse elements. Hence a dream of this kind, which makes its appearance in *different life-situations*, can be brought to the surface by various events in the dreamer's life. This is true of much of the *individual* stereotyped dreams, as of the *typical ones*, which occur in a similar fashion in the lives of most individuals (examination-dreams, flying dreams, etc.). Their *form* is determined by what is *common* to all human beings ; their full content and inherent *significance* is *individual*. This is proved also by the variability of associations, produced to such typical dreams. The examination dreams especially always have an individual feature, in that they deal in a recurrent manner with a certain school, class or subject. Stekel stated that in such dreams one never has to sit for an examination which one has *not* passed ; we dream only about examinations which we ourselves *did* pass successfully.[1] I dreamed in the past a few times that I had not done the work of the fifth form, that I had,

[1] Confirmed by Freud in his work *The Dream-Interpretation*.

therefore, not achieved the necessary qualification and justification for passing the matriculation and, consequently, the medical examination. In this dream I had my medical degree and I was afraid that, if discovered, I would have to make up the missed work. The historical background of this dream was, as follows : I was an external student, studied by myself, and had to pass an examination at the end of each year. When the preliminary examination in question was due (in June) I did not feel sufficiently prepared. I was also tired out, and reluctantly though, and afraid of " public opinion ", yet for safety I postponed the examination to September, the next possible date. If my memory serves me right, I passed with honours in all subjects at this later date. It seems really true, as Stekel suggests, that these dreams, occurring in critical moments of our lives, have the function of *comforting* us, for they reproduce the fear before an examination which *was passed*, i.e., an unfounded fear in the long run. It is clear that such examination dreams do *not* represent that particular examination as such, nor do they represent on different occasions the same complex. I have a few times tried to analyse more extensively such dreams in others ; I formed the impression that *no one* particular event of the historical past was hidden behind them, but that they represented the sum of many different contents. After all, the examination dreams are only one *special type of anxiety dream* ; and the central subject of our fears is essentially the integrity of our life in a biological, psychological and social sense. The examination dreams of a stereotyped kind show how some acquired experience-forms become firmly connected with the structure of the subconscious, and how much their individual content differs from their outer aspect. I want to emphasise particularly that, in my own case, when I went to the examination at the later date, I was in high spirits and had no fear at all with regard to the outcome ; so that the fear in my stereotyped dream could not be derived from the time of that examination. Perhaps, at the best, it could be related to the first occasion, when I did *not* venture the examination. Actually, the main idea in my dreams is that I did not go for the necessary examination at all (and not that I had failed and that someone might find this out). I did not experience this stereotyped dream in the last five years, though the present war with all its complications and dangers gave and continues to give reason enough for restlessness ; and though I have been faced during this period with a serious problem in my private life. Is this a sign of getting older, of mental stability in spite of disturbing events ; or is this a sign of inner resignation ; one does not fear any more whatever might come ? I do not dare to decide—I submit my observation to my readers and colleagues for them to think of, if they find it worthwhile. If fairly well analysed, one is enabled to see a great deal in one's own dreams, and what one interprets might be approximately right ; yet, presumably, the extent of what one is *not* able to see is far greater. . . .

There are, however, examination-dreams, which do not belong strictly to the described recurring type, and which are *not accompanied by anxiety of a greater degree.* Their content, and significance, is more specially coloured, than that of the above group. The following three dreams were dreamt in the *same night* ; each of them contains the *examination* motif :

87. (*a*) I am amongst other students, and we have to write a paper on " The Organization of Railways ". Since the topic is quite strange to all of us, we ask the examiner to outline briefly the single points. He complies with our wish. One of the fellow-candidates is *Mr. T.*, a friend from my childhood. . . .

(*b*) There is an examination ; I have to write a paper. Near by sits my *father*, who reads a letter and shows me something in it. I object to this, since the examiner might think that my father is helping me in composing the paper. . . .

(*c*) There is again an examination ; I cannot solve the mathematical problem and ask by a wink my *sister*, who apparently finished the task successfully, to give me some hint about the result. . . .

Associations : Mr. T. was the son of a strict, aristocratic *mother*, he was homosexual in consequence of a mother complex. In the dream he was about 18 years old. When he was 20, he had undergone a successful analytical treatment. The father of the dreamer was a talented lecturer, and was very much praised by the parents of Mr. T. Yet, he was always occupied by his scientific problems and could not get on with his *wife*, who was more realistically minded. She accused him of neglecting his family affairs. The sister of the dreamer was an egoistic person, who strove only for independence and an elegant life. She caused much trouble to

P

her *mother* and to the dreamer. The father, however, seemed to like her and to prefer her to the other children.

In the time of these dreams, my patient suffered very much from family affairs, and he felt that his plans for the future were too difficult to be solved. His mother tried to influence him to give up his intention of changing his profession and environment. He felt, accordingly, a certain sense of guilt towards his mother and sister, and he was aware that his sleeplessness and libidinous weakness was due to these facts.

It is easy to see how the motif of the *influencing mother* goes through all the three dream-scenes. To each of them there is one association, related to the mother. It seems that the last dream refers to the tendency to be independent, selfish, and to stick to his plan. This patient never had before, as far as his recollections go, examination dreams of the stereotyped and frightful character. This is, perhaps, indicative of the determined, independent way of his thinking and acting. He refuses in the dream to identify himself with his father, and is rather prepared to emulate his sister. In actual life, and in other respects, there was, on the contrary, a strong father-identification and a considerable antagonism towards the ways of his sister. True, during the analysis, both tendencies and attitudes lost much of their strength. He even consciously professed to giving up the abstract ideals of his father, and at the same time he felt more understanding for the neurotic selfishness of his sister in the past. *The above three dreams show clearly this psychoaffective change occurring in him.* He will probably continue in pursuing his aims.

(11) Somewhat different is the nature of the following stereotyped dream of a female patient :

88. I am sitting on a w.c. with the door bolted, or isn't it ?

The most important determining factor for this dream was the fact that, as a child, this patient had suffered from constipation, and had been given enemas against her will, by her paranoid mother, up to the age of 10 or 12 years. The father, in his position of authority, used to be present on these occasions. As an adult, this woman constantly administered an enema to herself, " in order to sleep better ". It should be pointed out that she was absolutely frigid, and although she got rid of her hysterical attacks (in which she used to fall on the floor) by the treatment which, unfortunately, did not last longer than three months,[1] no change was attained in her frigidity. She was 47 when she first came to see me. Four years later she went to Dr. Stekel, after her nervous complaints had re-appeared, though at rare intervals. (I sent her to him, as she had become a friend of my family and so it was not possible for me to take up analysis again.)[2] At this time these " toilet dreams " had ceased to occur in the second analysis, i.e., they had been actually eliminated by the earlier treatment. I also know that the enema-compulsion had lost much of its force. In this case the stereotyped dream was obviously influenced, even with regard to its manifest form, by an infantile, traumatic event, or rather by a series of such dramatic experiences. It contains the specific masturbation-phantasy of the patient, which enabled her at times to have a kind of orgasm. I had the impression that dreams of this patient were essentially stimulated more or less from the erogenous anus (organically stimulated dreams). I emphasise this because I want to offer reasons for the *strong hold* this type of dream has. I believe that all such stereotyped dreams have a definite, rather physical, " stimulus nucleus ". The remaining detailed content takes its origin from psychic sources, and is connected with the central stimulus by way of associations. I have pointed out elsewhere [3] that the formation of definite complexes (in the sense of classical psychoanalysis), i.e., of " verbalisable " contents, is facilitated by an organic stimulus-nucleus, acting as a ferment. The simplest example I can offer is perhaps a case of wash-compulsion I once had to treat, which was connected with fear from infection. In the anamnesis it was found that as a child the patient had to be forced to wash. I think that a child who has clean habits and yet has to be forced to wash is probably suffering from a *special sensitiveness of the skin against water*. Indeed, one *does* gain this impression in the case of many children. I mean actually to assert, then, that the nucleus of the washing and water complex in this case was somehow laid down organically. I would explain in a similar manner the great constancy of stereotyped dream motifs ; they are, as it were, " organic " parts of the

---

[1] At that time I was strongly influenced by the principle of short treatment advocated by Stekel ; yet one should be acquainted, too, with the principle of necessary " exceptions ".

[2] Vide the first case in Stekel's *Advances in Dream-Interpretation*.

[3] Lecture on " The choice of organ in the neurosis ", given to the Viennese Society for " Active Psychoanalysis ", 1936.

personality, because of the primarily organically stimulated nucleus they possess. This origin, however, need not restrict our analytical efforts at all, because, as explained above, a large number of modified contents become associated secondarily with the original complex.

A few additional remarks about this case of wash-neurosis might be of some interest. A great number of the dreams of this patient contained the motif of *water*. Frequently she dreamt about huge rivers, floods, endless seas, or of lesser quantities, of springs and water buckets. Several associations led to the father and two memories occurred to her repeatedly ; that she used to go *swimming* with him when she was a girl of ten to twelve, and that he had in the last years of his life a prostatic hypertrophy and suffered frequently from difficulties in *urination*. These motifs appeared in the dreams and associations more frequently and openly in the second half of the treatment. Only a very moderate therapeutic success was obtained, in so far as the extent of her restrictions (not to touch objects) and the time spent for washing, were considerably limited and her general behaviour and frame of mind became much more normal. My analysis lasted a year and was started after three years of previous illness. It could be established that when she was sixteen, a dog lifted her skirts and attempted to lick her legs ; after this event she felt the compulsion for a few months to wash thoroughly her genitals. Her recent illness started when she was 27, in the first year of her marriage, a few weeks after her father died. At first she washed only her hands when she touched anything in the house where she was employed, and where several artists, whom she suspected to have venereal disease, were wont to stay. Her husband—though really a fine type of man and also an artist—seemed not to keep pace with her lively temperament and it was he who had mostly to suffer from her very ramified neurosis. I do not want to dwell on this case ; yet I thought it deserved a brief description in connection with the dream motif mentioned.

(12) The group of typical dreams which occur in identical or similar form in most people, in so far as they contain the theme of *flying*, *floating* or *falling*, are very likely based on definite organic events. It has always been maintained that the self-perception of breathing and of the heart-beat, and the lack of sensation of pressure from the mattress during sleep

(hence the floating on air in dreams), are responsible for these kind of dreams. The dream in which one appears in the nude was similarly explained by the fact that there is a realisation of one's lying in bed without clothes.[1] For the *sudden fall-dream* I should hold the changing sleep-depths, together with the accompanying vasomotor processes, responsible. But in all these cases it has often been possible to show that the "content" was psychically overdetermined. I have found that some patients bring up more free associations to such dreams, others less or not at all. It is difficult to produce free associations to one's own " body " or bodily functions and properties. Perhaps introspective and self-observing individuals in general are more likely to produce a large number of associations to such typical " organic " dreams. This assumption is based only on a few single observations ; yet close connection with the " organ " of such dreams, and also the deep-rootedness of their content, might make.it understandable that people who are more aware of their " body ", overcome the difficulty in associating to such dreams.

Federn has argued that dreams of *flying* are erotically determined. The " going up " is supposed to signify erection.[2] I had no opportunity to observe and to investigate properly, cases which might definitely support this view ; but the possibility of its correctness has to be admitted. (In two cases I encountered dreams, occurring during erection, in which, repeatedly, weapons and sticks appeared ; in both cases these objects were in a perpendicular position.) Silberer has reported the following flying-dream, of a psychologically trained man, who had a pollution at the same time.

89. I am in a block of flats where I used to live when I was a child. I go up to the fourth floor, where I notice a trapeze-like apparatus. I get on to it and begin to swing to and fro ; this movement turns into *floating*. Thereupon the dizziness which troubled me at first vanishes. I float up and down rhythmically. . . .

---

[1] This explanation obviously obtained for the times when it was customary to wear loose-fitting night-shirts for sleeping apparel, and it was possible, therefore, for the sleeper to realise his relative nakedness, e.g., by apposition of his thighs. (Dr. T. Hart.)
[2] Quoted by Freud. The same author, in a later article, pointed out that irritations of the vestibular organ are the basis of such dreams ; we might add that every " psychogenic vertigo " felt in reality, originates from similar but more intensive " nervous irritations " of the same physiological apparatus.

The dreamer added that certain erotic memories were associated with that particular floor. This example definitely explains the relation between the content and the " container ". The connecting link between the floating-dream and its erotic content is, of course, the rhythmical nature of the excitement, which was experienced in a subliminal intensity in the genitals during sleep. But, as pointed out above, the "organic" basis of these dreams is indisputable. The following observations of Kimmins in his book on children's dreams, give full proof of this assertion.

" Under the general title of the kinæsthetic dreams we include the great variety of falling sensations, gliding, floating on air or water, often accompanied by loss of muscular and speech control. There are various explanations given of the cause of this type of dream, but, so far, no really satisfactory conclusion has been reached. From the present investigation it appears :

1. That children under the age of nine or ten years rarely experience it.
2. That from ten years of age it increases in frequency, fairly steadily, up to the age of seventeen or eighteen.
3. That well-fed children are more subject to it than those living under less favourable circumstances.
4. That regular institutional life tends to diminish this type of dream very considerably.
5. That deaf children scarcely ever have kinæsthetic dreams.
6. *That children who have had influenza or any type of malady* accompanied by high temperature are particularly susceptible to it (pp. 26–7).

" Dreams of this type occur only occasionally among children of eight and nine years of age ; *much more frequently among boys than girls.* It is at the age of ten that they form an important element in children's dreams, and from that age to fourteen they increase steadily. *Boys have more kinæsthetic dreams than girls, the proportion being ten to seven.* The gliding, floating and swimming elements are more common among girls, and the falling element among boys " (p. 63).

The difference observed between deaf and normal children, as well as the sex-differences at various ages and the influence of food, the living-standard in general, and of illness, suggest enough to the experienced and thinking medical man about the biological-physiological basis of this type of dream, even though we may not be in the position to give an exact account of the respective physiological background.

On the problem of *nude-dreams* the following should be said. Freud, consistent with his general views, reduces this type of dream to the infantile liking of the child to expose his body. The fact that such a tendency exists in the adult also cannot be doubted. But this does not exclude the earlier, more primitive explanation, given above (p. 213) as to the formative, frame-giving factor. The fact that such dreams are often accompanied by a painful emotion, even anxiety, and that such an element of painful embarrassment and anxiety is often felt in those allied dreams in which only a shoe-lace or a button is missing, severely curtails the general explanatory value of Freud's hypothesis. The fright in such dreams is not sufficiently explained by the sense of shame or *reaction* of the super-ego to the *exhibitory* tendencies. When I add that, according to the findings of the Viennese heart-specialist, Professor Braun, such dreams of embarrassment and also " nude-dreams " may indicate an incipient genuine angina pectoris, being therefore caused by disturbance of the circulation, then the scope of Freud's interpretation is, of course, still further reduced. But there is no doubt that from the psychoaffective infantile level the exhibitory tendency contributes the formative *basic factor.* I want only to draw attention here to the necessity of proper interpretation of the associated content, i.e., the utilisation according to each individual case.

As to the " inhibition-dreams ", earlier authors assumed that they originate in the perception of one's inhibited motility during sleep.[1] Federn, however, has argued that the organic nucleus of these dreams lies in the fatigued condition of the musculature. (Reverse parallelism is the psychogenic tiredness of many neurotics.) I can support his explanation, in so far as in two cases studied by me. I also could reduce the inhibition of motility implied in the dream-situation to actual tiredness. In one case the situation in the dream was that the dreamer felt that his legs were too *thin* and *weak* to enable him to mount a staircase. But in both cases the dream had a bearing upon real life-difficulties in which the dreamer found himself at that time. This was shown quite obviously by the fact that persons occurred in the dream who stood in close

[1] Cf. p. 228.

causative relation to his personal difficulties. In the first case there was among other worries a fear of getting sexually older (staircase $=$ intercourse !). It should be added that, according to Braun, such inhibition-dreams also may point to disturbances of the coronary circulation.

With regard to tooth-stimulus dreams, I could show similar conditions of dream-formation in one closely studied case. The patient as a young man dreamed very frequently that his teeth were falling out, dissolving and filling his mouth, whereupon he felt great embarrassment. After he ceased having remorses about his masturbation, according to his memory, he had not observed these dreams any more. His own explanation was in line with Freud's symbolic equation, which latter is in principle certainly correct, according to which a tooth might represent the male genitals, and the losing of the tooth symbolises the loss of sperms by masturbation (and perhaps the subsequent fear of having caused " castration " to himself.) But when I examined the case more closely, I discovered also that my patient had been suffering at that time a great deal from toothache. Thus the organic stimulus demanded this particular type of frame for the dream-content. The cessation of this dream type coincided with the cessation of the attacks of toothache, after my patient paid more attention to the care and dental treatment of his teeth. We do not want, of course, to cast any doubt on the psychological interpretation given by the dreamer ; I felt obliged to agree with him in view of the case history and the results of the analysis. But the *choice* of the tooth-dream, as a representation of his conflict, was certainly determined by his caries.

I have gone into detail in regard to these conditions, in order to confirm the interpreter in his work, and to show him the probable relationship between an organic event and the subsequent psychic content of the dream. Dreams dealing with the loss of teeth can, of course, also express other topics and problems ; for instance, the feared, or wished-for, death of a close relative, or the gradual giving up of convictions which have been firmly held as part of the ego-structure. The explanation of Freud, according to which the mechanism of displacement from below to above, gives the basis for the tooth-symbolism, applies of course only for the sexual interpretation given by him, but shows no bearing on the other mentioned symbolical possibilities. However, I think that in some cases where in the case history there is detectable a really marked castration-fear, the different fears of losing something dear and precious, might actually be linked up with the former complex, and the sexual symbolism might therefore be regarded as the form- and frame-giving basis, even where the more actual meaning refers to a quite different content.

(13) *The influence of bodily conditions and positions on the dream.* It is an indisputable fact that the particular position of the body and its individual parts might exert a considerable influence on the dream-material and on the elaboration of the dream-imagery. De Sanctis reported long ago that changing one's position during sleep changes the dream. I can confirm this from my own personal experience, though I could not notice essential changes of the content. The observations and records of Mourly Vold also show clearly that the actual position of one's limbs during sleep may be represented with fair accuracy in the dream. If one changes the position of the sleeper's limbs, then this movement may be incorporated into the dream in its actual form, or one may dream that one tried to perform that particular movement but could not carry it out. Sometimes, so Vold asserts, animals appear in the dream which, in their form, show some analogy to the position of the limb. Silberer also reports two cases [1] in which a particular position of the legs contributed to the dream-content. In the one, the simpler case, a certain position of the leg caused the hallucination of a similarly placed wooden log in the dream. In the second instance, which was so complicated that I shall extract only the " somatic relation " from it, the dreamer " was in a church with his feet in the fluting of a gothic pillar ; but he was at right angles to the pillar, i.e., in a recumbent position ". Actually, one of his legs lay under the other, at a right angle, when he awoke. We add another example :

90. I am lying and two women stroke my head, one on each side.

After awakening the dreamer remembers having stroked his child the evening before ; he also remembers the way his mother used to stroke his head while combing his hair. Only then did he notice that he had both his hands actually under his head. The influencing rôle of bodily conditions and

[1] Case 27.

positions seems to be not equally strong in every case of dreaming. Different kinds of investigations I carried out convinced me that there are marked individual varieties and even in the dream-life of the same individual the bodily position and condition does not appear recognisable in the dream-image with regularity.[1] I cite three dreams experienced during strong urinary urge by three different people :

> **91.** I am in the bed : my friend Reverend F. comes to me and wants to know whether my shirt is *wet* or dry ; it appears to be dry. Then he comes once more and examines me again ; the night dress is still not wet. . . .

Association : Two days before, the mentioned reverend made an ironical remark as to the rare occasions on which the dreamer attended church. This memory explains the motif of searching. The allusion to the urination-urge is, however, recognisable.

> **92.** The dreamer sees a colleague of his and speaks only reluctantly to him. The latter explains something about his own brother and says repeatedly, " He told me several times he does not yet want to die ".

Association : " The whole dream situation was *unpleasant* and I understood that my brother fights against his suicidal tendencies." The unpleasantness of the situation, and also the fight against an impulse, obviously originates, in part at least, from the urge which has to be controlled. However, it is difficult to deny the psychogenic origin of the dream content. The dreamer had, in fact, experienced suicidal tendencies in the period when the dream occurred.

> **93.** I cannot read the last line of a typewritten page ; *it is painful not to be able* to discover the connection of the text. I try again and again. Awakening under strong urination-urge. . . .[2]

The prone position of the dreamer seems also to become conscious in some dream experiences, probably only in superficial sleep. One of my acquaintances dreamed :

> **94.** I am expecting a telegram (I was actually expecting one that morning) ; suddenly a messenger boy comes in and behaves in a most familiar manner ; he lies down on my bed, but at the same time he remains at the door, as if he

---

[1] See pp. 227–8.   [2] Cf. Ch. II, dream 12, and p. 34.

were just coming in. While I am awakening I feel as if *I were the person lying in the bed.*

The associations to the boy led to the problem of suicidal tendencies connected with an insoluble conflict ; the expected wire had some bearing upon this question. The messenger boy represented therefore *Death* ; and his playful behaviour, and his near and distant position, symbolised the bipolar atti-tude of the dreamer to such a serious plan. (Suicide implies the *identity* of the killer and the killed person. Similarly, the dreamer felt that he and the boy, lying on the bed, are the same person.) Besides, there were recollections about jealousy and *homosexually* coloured ideas of inferiority.

Well known is a " comfort-dream " once cited by Freud. A medical student had one morning to get up and go to the clinic ; he went to sleep again and saw himself lying in a hospital bed as a patient. He said to himself, " Since I *am* in the hospital anyway, I might as well stay in bed."

(14) The psychotherapist, especially if he is used to employ the " active and intuitive " method of interpretation of Stekel, might often ask himself in the course of his professional life whether he does not run too great a risk of making mistakes in looking upon the dream in all its parts and aspects as a pure psychic construction, and in drawing conclusions readily from these details. Here is one example to illustrate the funda-mental difficulty involved. A man, who as far as could be ascertained used to cross, or to bend, his legs during sleep, dreamed :

> 95. I see a pointed hill in which two aeroplanes have buried their noses. They stand at *right angles* to each other.

The patient interpreted this *right angle* himself, by giving the following association : " Yesterday a friend told me I could live only by fixed rules ; indeed, any compromise is difficult for me. I look at everything from the *right angle*." As I had the impression that the dream contained much more, viz., the representation of his endopsychic state (he had consciously approached his actual conflict from *two* aspects, but he had not discovered the deeper connection between them), I asked him intuitively whether the two machines had *touched*. He was taken aback and said, " No, they were separate. I myself found that strange, even in the dream ". Of course, if we bear in mind similar accidents in reality, it would have been rather surprising if the two 'planes *did* really touch in a geo-metrically exact manner ; yet, as I have just said, the true dream-content represented the two insights which had not coalesced into the required, sensible unity. Hence he was actually justified in being surprised within the dream at the failure of the machines to touch. His being astonished signifies the subconsciously " felt " knowledge that the aeroplanes are only symbols of attitudes. As at that particular stage of his analysis he was not yet mature for such a disclosure, I had simply to confirm his—also correct, though not " self-con-tained "—interpretation, and said, " The failure of the two machines to touch reflects actually your incapacity to *compromise*."

But we must return to the problem we posed above and ask ourselves ; could not the dream-image be reduced quite simply to the position of the limbs ? Or perhaps to his two hands clasping the corner of the eider-down while asleep ? There is a certain probability in favour of the first supposition, viz., that his legs were at right angles to each other. How then, does it come about that both his and my " meaningful " interpretation appear so well in agreement with the dream-image ? Is it an accident ? Are our interpretations strained ? Are they mere poetic constructions, even more than the dreams themselves ? Those who have encountered convincing cases, where such an intuitive idea made possible an important therapeutic step forward, those who have had the satisfaction of obtaining later confirmation for an idea at first only vaguely " felt ", will say, with justification, " Better two unfounded interpretations (as long as a thoughtless or premature com-munication to the patient *does not do therapeutic harm*) than one missed opportunity through a too critical proceeding ". Fortunately the situation is not as precarious as that. We must ask ourselves why the particular position and condition of the body does not always find its recognisable reflection in the dream-image, not even when it becomes disturbing, irritating, and leads to awakening ? And why the great individual differences in the dream-representation of such universal bodily positions ? The transformation of a somatic sensation into a psychic construction is a fact. I mean by that not only the reproductive, pictorial dramatisation of the physical stimulus in the dream-image, but also the genuine, inherent connection of the somatic stimulation with other subconscious and half-conscious material. I am convinced that *somatic-stimulus-sources really do enrich the psychoaffective contents and states* ; otherwise several facts regarding psychophysical relations would *not* be intelligible. Rather than be vague, I shall express my opinion and hypothesis in a, perhaps, slightly imaginative form in connection with the cited example, in saying : Possibly the crossing of the legs, and the inconvenience created thereby, have actually strengthened the respective complex of the " difficult compromise-formation ", at least during sleep. (I think the mental significance of the self-perception in sleep is actually different from that in waking, and also that the influencing intensity of the complexes is deeper in sleep or in day-dreaming, because the " attention of life " is turned away from reality.) If that is so, are we not fully justified in interpreting the dream-element, even if primarily or mainly stimulated by somatic-physical events ?

The following example is simple and therefore all the more illustrative. A young man, who is being treated because of sexual difficulties, comes to the conclusion that he lost his libidinous freedom largely through the warnings of his mother against girls and rash marriage. But he was *not* fully conscious of the following fact—and could not appreciate at first its importance, even after his attention was drawn to it—that by listening up to the age of 25 to his parents' intercourse with excitement and final orgasm, he had become *fixated very strongly on this libidinous situation*.[1] Thus, the mother became an inhibiting factor in *two ways*. When I found that he was not yet prepared for this aspect of the problem, I did not touch upon it for weeks and waited till he himself would come to speak of it. This period of growing analytically mature finally came and was heralded by the following dream :

> **96.** My brother Paul discovers my mother, frozen, underneath a tree ; then I come and try to revive her.

No free associations were produced. He mentioned only incidentally that he had been particularly *cold* that night. It is not, then, possible to overlook the contributory part played by the disturbing cold in the formation of the dream-experience. The psychological interpretation admits of various formulations. One might see in the dream-image a disguised allusion to erotic plays (attempts at " reviving " = as a sexual

[1] Cf. Ch. III (31).

symbol) ; or one might think that the patient begins to
" revive " his mother-complex, i.e., to become conscious of
it, in accordance with the aims of the analyst. (The brother
Paul had shown to the patient a great deal of understanding ;
his image sometimes took the place of the understanding
analyst in transference dreams.) In any case, the allusion to
the mother-complex of the patient is rather obvious. When
I add that in the acts to which the patient had listened, the
mother had behaved rather *coldly* and with reserve, so that the
father had to persuade her ; when we know, from the admissions
of the patient, that this annoyed him, because thereby his own
orgasm was delayed, then the " freezing " of the mother in
the dream is easily explained ; even without taking into
account the first interpretation, viz., that the patient is beginning only now to "*feel*" the repressed complex.

What I want to demonstrate here, is the close unity between
physical and psychic dream-stimulation, and the *congruence of
" mental " content, inherent in both types of stimulus.*[1] *I think that
we are not justified in brushing aside the assumption that the feeling of
the cold has awakened the psychic content of the respective complex in
the dream* : at least this is possible and indeed probable. We
may conceive of the dream-forming process in the somewhat
following way :

The depth-psychic analytical process has arrived at the
mother-fixation complex, which begins to become more capable of consciousness. The " feeling of cold " then stimulates
and intensifies *that* part of the complex-content, which is connected with the relative coldness of the mother when approached
by her husband. The actual attempt to snuggle closer into
the blankets during sleep may have touched upon the memory
of my patient's displeasure at his mother's cool refusal, because
that disturbed his own de-tumescence and " emotional
warmth ". As a result, the dream emerges in which the
brother represents the analyst, but, at the same time, the
father, and functionally also the progressively unravelling
analytical process. The patient " feels " more and more the
complex in question ; he " revives " the mother in himself—
at the same time he revives his libido in connection with the
figure of his mother. He was not told this interpretation ;
yet he began spontaneously to talk about the very same theme

---

[1] Compare Ch. X, where the " affectenergetic " identity of both stimuli is
pointed out.

the next day. After one week he recalled that in his masturb-
atory phantasies he used to place his partners into the bed of
his parents. This, I believe, is the finishing touch necessary
to make the interpretation convincing. Two weeks later he
was advised by me to imagine intercourse with his fiancée
before going to sleep. At first success was only superficial
because the revived mother complex made it even more
difficult than previously. Finally, however, full therapeutic
success was obtained ; the clever behaviour of his wife (he
had. married) greatly facilitated it.

(15) It is established that somatic sensations, like dyspepsia,
bronchial trouble, pains, etc., are dramatised and personified
in the dream. It is also certain, on the other hand, that
affective states call forth certain organic reactions which are
relatively constant in each individual. Thus the psychosomatic unity, on which recent authors have laid so much
stress, is shown from both these aspects to be a reality.

From here it is only one further step to the assumption made
above, viz., that organic sensations strengthen not merely simple
elementary affect-qualities, but also intensify, actualise, elaborated and ramified complex-contents.[1] The various organic
functions have always signified something to the human mind
(the heart = goodness ; the liver = anger and envy ; the
breath = life ; the right side = that which is right and good,
etc.) ; and it seems to me unjustified to restrict to only a few
instances such " symbolic signification " of organs, organic
functions, positions and conditions. *For the deep consciousness,
everything " organic " has a meaning and a psychoaffective content.*
For this reason we may confidently interpret, or try at least
to approach the understanding of, every dream-image. In
actual practice we shall, of course, never attribute too much
importance and argumentative value to one single anxiety
dream, for instance, without having studied thoroughly the
complete case history in all its parts and aspects, and without
having compared that dream with the rest of the dream-
material at our disposal. We are now convinced more than
ever that there exists always a *conscious link* to any therapeutically important *subconscious complex*. I have tried to
investigate the problem of the justified ability of dream-
interpretation in connection with my own dreams and. those
of others, for years. I am quite convinced that the usual

[1] Cf. p. 123–4.

way of "psychological interpretation" is well founded; though at the same time I had to come to the conclusion—more than other contemporary dream-psychologists—that *all our dreams contain to a very great extent so-called somatic material.*[1] We can, however, during practical work either neglect this latter contribution to dream-formation, or assume, as suggested in this work, that somatic events *do* influence and strengthen complexes; to a considerable extent, however, only during sleep, i.e., the period of dreaming. I want to add two carefully studied examples to this point. A man who suffered upon occasions from the feeling of sexual and general insufficiency, once dreamed following an auto-erotic act, after which he felt sick:

> **97.** I see Mr. B. eating something greedily, but he seems to think that the food is *too greasy.* His wife stands near me and talks about her musical concert. Then I see two small bananas, each of which has a thick, black worm in it. I wake up feeling replete.

Associations : Mr. B. is very fond of eating well and abundantly; he is an egoist. So is his wife, to an even higher degree. She is a pianist and lives only for her music. She loves her children, but lets others care for them. The day before the dream my patient had thought of this family, of the children and their well-being, and wondered whether they were far from bombed Paris. In the evening of the same day he had given his own child a banana, to supply him with the necessary vitamins. This child had lately caused him certain worries, and he was afraid that his work and life-struggle in general might be made more difficult in consequence; he felt that his child might become his enemy. The day before the dream he himself was suffering from lack of appetite, and thought with disgust of greasy food. . . .

All these ideas cover sufficiently the individual dream-elements and also the deeper dream-content. The patient's incidental dyspepsia is alluded to twice—by the unpalatable

---

[1] K. Leonhard (1939) in a small book on dreams tried to show that the different categories of dream-elements originate always from the waking life; yet they re-appear in the dream after various intervals. Colours, sounds, pleasurable and disagreeable impressions have, according to this author, a different latency and incubation period. He concludes that there is, therefore, no justification at all for psychoanalytical utilisation of dreams. We need not argue against this conclusion; practical experience disproves it. The regularity of the latency-interval may, however, prove stimulating to further investigation on the intimate conditions of the *affect-regulative mechanism,* the existence of which had been suggested by nearly all my articles on psychology. (*Die Gesetze des Träumens, Thieme, Leipzig.*)

food and the loathsome worms. The dreamer had the definite feeling that this was an organically stimulated dream. On the other hand, one can hardly overlook the problem of his child, alluded to through the egoistical, easy-going parents in the dream. The banana, with the disgusting worm, pointed unmistakably, at the same time, to the disturbed parent-sentiment ; and also, of course, to his sexual difficulties. One might say, as is usual, that somatic and psychic sources have come together in the formation of the dream. But this is only a working hypothesis ; the homogeneous coalescence of these two groups of contents has been carried out too thoroughly to allow of such a simple view. The two parents (one of them eating the indigestible food), and also the bananas with the worms—both motifs together express both elements, viz., the father-child conflict on one hand and the dyspepsia on the other hand. One cannot help saying that *the dyspepsia has added an intensifying contribution to the respective mental conflict, and has so aided in the creation of the conflict-dream.* Once we get accustomed to this unitary conception of dreams, this fashion of looking upon the individual dream-images seems quite natural and logical. Just as a conflict-situation, or rather the accompanying affective disturbance (parapathia), *can* call into being or intensify an attack of dyspepsia, similarly and reversely an organic event of this kind *can* very well lend emphasis during sleep to a " disturbing complex ". As we have seen in an earlier chapter, the normal organic functions present a constant basic element for the formation of dreams. It is surely obvious that dysfunctions of the same organs, use the same organo-psychic reflex paths in exerting their psychic influences, and so are in a position to strengthen the mental complexes.[1] The theory propounded here does not lessen the justification of interpreting dreams ; on the contrary, it enhances it. For we do *not* believe in some accidental and " irregular " mingling of organic and psychic elements ; but only *in one unitary dream content, i.e., the psychoaffective one.* We may refer back to the chapter on the biological function of dreaming, where we attempted to show the essential similarity and energetic equivalence of these two dream-sources. *This latter principle too, appears to be one basic presupposition for any dream-interpretation.*

The background and process of formation of the following

---

[1] Cf. also dreams 14 and 72.

dream could have been more thoroughly studied ; the dreamer is a medical student who is interested in physiological and psychological research, is a good observer too, and has the faculty of producing easily free associations. The day previous to the dream he *played football and was very tired.* During the following night he frequently awoke, restless, and felt muscle-strain. He also experienced a *"fulness in his stomach"*, though he went to bed without supper, because he had no appetite, owing to his fatigue. He smoked, however, ten cigarettes within an hour before falling asleep, for him an unusual amount for such a short spell. The next morning he was supposed to do an urgent writing job, which work he considered boring, and which he had postponed for several days from inner resist-ance. These were the " disturbing factors " preceding his sleep and his dream, as far as they could be established.

> **98.** There was in the dream a large sheet of paper, full-written, in the middle of which he saw a figure indicating a *"footnote"*. Here the page opened in some way into a *pouch*. This was similar to a *gastric pouch* in the well-known experi-ment of Pavlov, who divided by operation the stomach of a dog into a larger and a smaller part, creating thereby a miniature stomach beside the main cavity. In the dream, then, he had the impression that it is not right that the bigger part of the sheet should communicate with the smaller, minia-ture stomach-cavity, instead of the larger one.

Free associations : *Stomach, my father suffered from ulcer.* Pre-viously he suffered too, from rheumatic pains in his legs and was often *tired after a walk.* He seemed to suffer much from the sexual coolness of his wife. *Vagina, similar to the pouch in the dream.* (A break of several minutes in producing associations.) Quarrel between father and mother. He threatened with divorce. The children cried, the mother seemed to be frightened. She became quiet. Essentially both were cultured individuals, with an ethical outlook. I see father without shoes and stockings, as if he had *sore feet.* The " footnote " in the dream had the figure 1. Father wanted me to be a first-class scientist. He was conservative (so was Pavlov), yet he was fond of modernism in thinking. I am lately progressive, nearly communistic ; I feel a bit guilty, I could hardly reply to him if called to account. Yet I think he could understand my craving for love if he knew, because of his suffering. I read once, that some young people have inguinal and scrotal pains together with weak *feet*. The reason for this syndrome was not explained in the book.

The close bearing of the recollected material upon the manifest dream is obvious. Interesting is the relationship between the " footnote " and the repeated theme of " foot trouble " and fatigue. However, the dream event contains more obviously the motif " stomach ", than that of the tired legs and feet. But according to the associations, the pouch represents also the vagina ; though, of course, the allusion to the lack of appetite is not less obvious. As is well known, the experiments of Pavlov mentioned, dealt with the *psychic aspect of appetite and acid secretion*. I knew from the analysis, that the dreamer refrained from sexual activity before marriage, owing to ethical considerations. He was engaged, and his fiancée lived far away. . . . He would not be unfaithful. He thought that his *appetite* and general health would increase after marriage. . . .

I think the cited details allow the following conclusion : *The somatic condition enters the manifest dream in a recognisable fashion when its " psychoaffective content " connects manifestly with the " psychic content " creating the dream in question.* In the above case the stomach seems to carry a libidinous significance ; not only as a dream symbol, but actually, in the sense as explained above. So seem to have acquired the legs and feet a psycho-affective content, related to the sexual conflict of the dreamer, though only in a fashion not quite easily expressible in waking thoughts and words. See the supposed but not clearly explained relation between flat feet and inguinal pain.

I think, therefore, that if the somatic condition does not appear in the dream manifestly, it is so because its " psychoaffective content " is of such a kind, which is not capable of being thought and verbalised ; its cathexis is, however, present and active behind the dream. The free associations might hint from afar at such a content ; but they indicate only approximately the spheres of complexes in question. *The bodily condition in its fullness—normal and abnormal processes included—is nevertheless present and active in the dream-event.*

It has not avoided the attention of Freud, that organ-stimuli, whether of a normal intensity, or beyond the physiological threshold, appear recognisable only rarely in dreams. In his opinion, all physical dream-sources carry only an incidental (sleep-disturbing) significance ; and his explanation of the above problem is in line with his general conception.

He thinks that any organ sensation is being woven into the
dream picture, if it is suitable to serve as a constituent of that
dream which is going on independently. He analyses, for
instance, one of his dreams, in which he first quickly bounds up
the steps, incompletely clad. He meets the maid from the
house and suddenly, from embarrassment, he is rooted to the
spot and cannot move. He rightly points out that the actual
muscular immovability, prevailing during sleep, cannot itself
account for the dream-motive in question, since in the previous
scene he was able even to jump. So in his opinion the intrapsychic embarrassment, due to his exhibitionistic tendencies,
employs the sensation of being unable to move during sleep.
(I think this is the meaning of his explanation.)

This exposition is certainly true, *but it is probably so in a deeper
sense.* We explained, that organic conditions in fact do carry
and intensify complexes, mental contents, and it is not only
a formal and incidental contribution which they offer to the
dream-work. Provided that his dream deals, in fact, with
infantile exhibitionistic tendencies, the childish, easy way of
" bounding up " the steps, might belong to the same attitude,
and so there is even an intrinsic connection between both
dream events. The lying undressed in bed, might have
aroused infantile recollections and re-activated infantile attitudes in general, by virtue of the regressive mechanism at work
during sleep. The lying position in its different aspects might,
therefore, easily carry at the same time the different motifs,
i.e., mobility and immobility, appearing in the dream story.
This explanation, however, is probably not " the central
interpretation ". We have followed only the suggestion of the
dreamer. (Cf. *The Interpretation of Dreams*, Ch. V.)

It is obvious that *we* do not assume a fixed psychoaffective
content associated with the different organs and their functions. In human mental life in general, there is at the same
time a certain constancy and a continuous metamorphosis,
according to the requirements of life. The same holds probably of the psychoaffective processes pertaining to the somatic
organisation of personality.

(16) Though this book cannot deal with detailed aspects of
practical interpretation, it has given on several occasions, in
different connections, useful hints. Similarly, I should like
here to add, briefly however, an important point indicating
something not well enough known to many psychotherapists.

In certain cases, and especially in certain periods of the illness and treatment, when there seems no near prospect of improvement, no immediate prospect of disclosing the deeper background of the overt symptomatic state, when the whole thinking, associating of the patient is dominated by his complaints, most of the dreams are not capable of being analytically utilised. *They represent actually only the described subjective state,* from which the patient suffers at that given period, without disclosing to a considerable degree anything of the complexes lying behind the surface of symptoms. One should not take very great pains to go deeper into such dreams ; one should rather try to guess what they do *not* contain openly. Two examples of this kind :

> 99. I go upstairs and see suddenly a cat running across ; I get frightened, I have to stop. . . .

The patient suffers from agoraphobia, from neurotic heart-attacks, and cannot even walk upstairs when her anxiety takes the form of an intensified paroxysm. There are many factors to explain her state. The father is a drinker and tried to make love to his daughters ; the mother has a lover ; she herself is married to a man with a strange character.[1] It is, however, obvious for me that the dream above *expresses merely the dramatised symptom.* No useful gain can be achieved by letting the patient produce associations.

Another instance :

> 100. We are at home, everything seems to be funny ; there is a noise and I should like to leave the room. . . .

Here also the dream-image gives expression essentially to the neurotic state, which consisted in depressions and the general feeling of incapacity. The desire to get rid of all the inhibitions is also stressed by the dream.

As to the theoretical explanation of these analytically " useless ", superficial dreams, different possibilities present themselves. First, it might be that the disguising process is carried out to an extremely strong degree, so that practically the dream does not betray anything. The second possibility is that there is a kind of annulment ; the subconscious refuses to deal with the complexes, they are pushed into an encapsulated " corner " of the waking thinking and so are not available either to the dream world or to the clear realisation of consciousness. Such

[1] Cf. dream 80.

a mechanism was described by Stekel as existing in several cases of compulsive neurosis, where certain traumatic experiences were not really repressed, but annulled as described. He says, " they are pushed into the day-dreams and have to be guessed by the analyst ".[1]

For the more general dream-problem discussed now, I should, however, prefer a different conception. I think that in such cases there is a marked degree of repression, or rather a *considerable split-between the pathogenic deep levels* and *the conscious " suffering " surface* ; consequently, even the conceptual dreaming-process does not reach the usual depths, and reflects and represents only events of higher levels. This fact might also be cited in favour of the statement made in Ch. II. (2), *that the dreaming sphere is not the deepest Id, and as is seen, it might in certain stages of neurosis be " lifted " even to a higher psychic level.*

(17) The process of dreaming is at all events congruent with the total of the psychoaffective life. For the practical purpose of dream-interpretation, however, only the *remembered dream-images* come within consideration. It is a general assumption that the dream-content is closely associated with those conscious and subconscious mental processes, which constitute the basis and background of our patient's disturbed condition., However, closer observation compels us to re-view the problem of the relationship obtaining between dreams and psychic processes, and to modify the general character of the above assumption.

The previously discussed cases represent only *one* possibility where the congruity between the remembered dreams and the supposed deep psychic processes, seems to be lacking in a similar way. Schilder pointed first to the fact that melancholic patients of the clinic not infrequently dream that they are well, happy, and staying at home under the normal conditions prevailing previous to their illness. The dream-content consists chiefly of such trivial elements related to normal everyday life. (H. Deutsch similarly found that melancholics, if one succeeds in inducing them to produce free associations, recollect chiefly pleasurable memories, without, however, recognising the pleasure-quality of such associations.) Schilder concluded that the faculty of pleasure-experiencing is, to a certain degree, retained in the melancholic. However, the apparent contrast is remarkable. It is obvious that such dreams do *not* give expression to the suffering mental " system ",

[1] Cf. Ch. II, p. 67.

and neither to possible complexes, responsible for, or related to, the illness.

In melancholia the function of "self-experiencing" appears to be impaired. Yet, on the other hand we suggest in the present work that dreaming is an intensified ego-experience. There is only one, though simple, answer. The ego-feeling of the waking state and the ego-experience, by means of objectification and dramatisation as occurring in dreaming, are *two* related, complementary processes, *but they are of two kinds*. The *one* function might be grossly impaired, and the other one still in part retained. That this latter is, however, not fully intact in melancholia, is indicated by the intense sleeplessness, from which such patients suffer. Sleeplessness implies, of course, he exclusion of the dreaming-process.

Melancholia in general is not an object of psychoanalytic therapy. But similar discrepancies, as here, are to be found in neuroses. Some of the patients dream that their complaints do not exist ; that the agoraphobic walks freely ; the phobic is not afraid of that thing, which in waking, arouses his anxiety-reactions ; the impotent has no inhibitions (especially remarkable when he intercourses in the dream with the same person, in relation to whom he is in life impotent) ; and more similar. Most of the patients, however, do show in their dream, at least to a certain degree, that symptom for which they are treated.

In addition, we not infrequently meet individuals, too, who are *not* patients, and who dream mostly only about one [1] aspect of their life, and never, or only rarely, about the multitude of occurrences in their waking state. There is no doubt that there are individuals, and certain conditions and phases in patients, where there exists certainly a considerable degree of incongruity between the field encompassed by their dreams, and their total intrapsychic world. I think there is a pressing need for investigating this relationship on a larger scale ; only in possession of certain conclusions from a large material, will the utilisation of dreams in psychotherapy become a really reliable instrument, employed and relied upon only there, and in such extent, where there is presumably a prospect of its usefulness.[2]

Since the relative distinctness and independence of the produced *dream-images* from the *dreaming-process* seem to be

[1] This is not to be mistaken for cases where all dreaming occurs in terms of "professional" elements. (See Ch. VI (6) and (7).) [2] Ch. XII (21).

a fact, we may conclude that the biological need for the constant dreaming-process on one hand, and the additional need for producing the scenic, recollectable dream-images on the other, are neither fully parallel.[1] We may, therefore, at any rate, conceive the *dreaming-process* as embracing the total of the psychoaffective life ; and besides, realise that, at times, the material contained in the conceptualised, formed *dream-images*, takes its origin from only a limited field of psychoaffective happening. From this it follows, that the degree of significance for the analysis of dreams is variable, according to different individuals, stages of their illness, stages of the treatment, etc.

As to the significance of dreams in which the neurotic patient appears without his complaints and symptoms, this constitutes in general an indication of a good prognosis to a certain degree.[2] It is surely *so*, if the dreams of a patient acquire this character in the course of treatment. The " well-being dreams " of the melancholic, are probably also indicative of a good prognosis, as to final recovery. It is a not infrequent experience, that such patients recover after several months, or even one or two years, suddenly, overnight, from a symptomatically grave condition, without showing first the process of gradual improvement. This indicates that the self-healing process was all the time in operation, though overtly not recognisable. The more frequent are the dreams of the kind mentioned, the more probable it seems that the condition strives towards normal health.

(18) To bear in mind the difficulties, the actual impossibility, of interpreting every dream and each detail of any given dream, is in fact as much part and as fundamental a principle of our conception regarding this field as is the knowledge of all the positive rules guiding the practical and feasible act of interpretation and utilisation of dreams. In the course of our expositions we have repeatedly pointed out the discrepancy and incongruity regarding the quality and extent existing between the world of dreaming and that of waking thought. The substantial degree of transformation of experiences and thoughts into dream-material has been illustrated by the " reaction-dreams ",[3] and similarly by the differently structured urinary dreams.[4] One further point should be added here. Minute self-observation clearly shows that some, mostly

[1] Cf. p. 177.   [2] Cf. Ch. VIII (4).   [3] Cf. Ch. III.   [4] Cf. p. 218.

unpleasant, dreams seem closely connected with the fact of minor, yet disturbing, inconveniences of physical nature, experienced by the sleeping and dreaming person. Cold or heat in the bedroom, the pressure of creased bed-clothes, an inconvenient position of the limbs, sometimes the dim knowledge of having to get up soon for some duty, and similar factors, seem to account for dream-experiences, the content of which has no apparent bearing upon the actual irritation ; yet after this disturbing moment or factor has ceased to act, the previous dream might disappear entirely, or change its unpleasant features into a more smooth character. A man staying overnight in a place for the sake of fire-watching, spent a few hours in bed in his clothes, uncovered by blankets. The unusual situation rendered his sleep restless, he could not feel quite at ease, though his drowsiness and fatigue did not allow him to get up, to undress, and to cover. Continuously a dream appeared in which :

> **101.** A man whom he knew as a child, was singing on the stage, clumsily gesticulating, and another person, apparently young and tall, but *not shaved*, stood by and was supposed to be the musical author of the show. . . .

The acting person was in real life a book-seller, a kind but not very clever, short-sighted and plain-looking man, who could not be even imagined as a singer or actor. The composer reminded him of a singer in a church choir, whom the dreamer also had not seen for about 15 years. The previous night before going to bed he thought of having *dark superfluous hairs in his ears*, which annoyed him. The other person of the dream reminded him of the fact that a plain-looking man has to be satisfied with marrying a plain-looking girl. Our dreamer was at that time in love with a nice-looking girl. . . . This was all that could be related to his present problems and condition. After about two hours struggling in a half-sleeping state, he pulled off his trousers and crawled under the blankets and, though continuing to dream, the *unpleasant character of the dream, and also the appearance of the dream-figures changed.* We cannot but consider the dream in its first form and content as expressing the inconvenient bodily condition, the acting figures and their external deficiencies being adequate to the unpleasant subjective state of the sleeper. We are dealing here with a kind of *reaction dream*, chiefly related to the physical inconvenience. The choice of the particular dream-elements, in this case too, has been determined by memories and individual problems, pointing to the past and the present. However, it seems obvious that in this dream the dreamer experienced his own ego, the present condition of his " self ", which latter is in fact always a product of the whole individual past and present ; but surely and first of all, such dreams are related to the *condition of the psychosoma during sleep.* Actually, we hold the opinion that *all dreaming is essentially a mode of self-experiencing ; all the memories and deposits of past experiencing have become ego-parts and appear as such in the dreams.* What has been said about the biological status of dreaming in relation to affect-metabolism is, in fact, only a partial aspect of this broader concept of " self-experiencing ".

Bearing all that in mind, we are now enabled to look deeper into the difficulties of dream-interpretation. When the physician listens to the normal or *pathognomical* breath sounds, he utilises certain physical qualities of conditions, obtaining in the respiratory system during its functioning. Yet, it is more than natural that the essential rôle of the air, and secretion in the pulmonary vesicles does not imply the diagnostic aspect ; all those sounds are not existent just in order to be heard by ausculation. It is, therefore, obvious that those physical qualities, by reason of which these sounds are being detectable and examinable, constitute *not* the essential feature, and even less the complete content, of what occurs in the bronchioli and alveoi, when air and secretion are moving in them. The audibility of these events is an additional, side-line character of them.

It is somewhat similar with the dreams. We have found that the dreaming process is probably part of the affect-regulative processes ; we have found also that the essential function of dreaming is, even more surely, the ego-experiencing, in fulfilment of a corresponding biological human need. The diagnostic utilisation of the dream-material is an artificial act of human intelligence, comparable to ausculation.[1] True, any concept of self-experiencing implies intrinsically some kind of " self-conceiving " and " self-understanding ". If the dreaming actually aims primarily at self-experiencing, so is this undoubtedly carried out by dramatisation and personification of the ego-tendencies and ego-conditions ; this means implicitly an "understandable mode" of the ego-experiencing. Hence,

[1] Cf. p. 177.

there is something in the essential character of the dreaming-process, even taken as a psychobiological process, which facilitates the meaningfulness and "interpretability" of the resulting and recollected dream-image. But the fact remains that the point of view of the interpreter, and the essence of the complicated and total process of ego-experiencing, lie on two distinct levels. Hence, the lack of congruity between the true extent of dreaming and the interpretable part of the recollected image appears in any case only natural. It is obvious that the interpreted content is frequently only a conclusion, but not *that* content which constitutes the genuine dreaming-events. It is, as if we take an expression as a noun, though in the actual sentence that word was used as a verb. Our dream-interpretation aims at the understanding of the waking personality, of its feeling and thinking—conscious and unconscious—and of the mode of its behaving. Yet, this dreaming is actually a different category of life-event, it is a psychoenergetic event, resulting in "ego-experience", though its constituents are mental elements of the waking state. Consider as an analogy the categorical difference between "subject" as an adjective, as a noun, as a verb, and finally, in its use in the form "subjective". The linguist is aware of the close association of the different forms, yet who could deny the marked categorical differences obtaining between them?

What we interpret is, therefore, mostly a new structure of the interpreting mind. I should like to illustrate the supposed facts by an imagined analogy. But first I shall quote a dream I heard from a patient.

> **102.** He saw first in a corner of a room a couple speaking; then apparently in another room, which appeared to be distant from the first and on a different level, he saw a bookcase; then it seemed to him as if time and space would part both previous fragments from a third scene. He saw and heard the *well-known* Lisa Fuchsova playing a Mozart piece. The listeners sat in their chairs, but at the same time the *hall was empty* [1]; the dreamer saw simultaneously the above-mentioned two scenes. . . .

The subjective unity of the dream-experience was main-

[1] This means: His psyche is fully occupied by "the melody of his central complex", symbolised here by the play of the "well-known" Czech pianist. Well-known = He was afraid that some people could discover the reason of his neurotic troubles. There is nothing else at present within the horizon of his interest; "the hall is empty". This refers perhaps also to his wish that no one should gain insight into his difficulties. "The listeners sat in their chairs, but at the same time the hall was empty."

tained and still the described gaps in space and time were experienced. This dream-description gave me the following idea. Let us imagine a complicated picture, a scene full of details. Some parts of the painting are done with the usual paints ; other parts with a kind of ultravisible material, which could be seen only by a specially constructed apparatus. In applying the analogy : the original and total dream-experience contains some fragments, accessible not only to the dreaming-ego, but also the conceiving mind ; the bulk of the dream-experience is effectuated only in the specific mode of dreaming. Those conceivable fragments carry at the same time this specific dreaming-character ; their conceivable quality is, for certain reasons, superposed upon their essential character.[1] The homogeneity of the dream-total is so present ; and certain fragments are at the same time conceivable and capable of being remembered and interpreted. The gaps in the dream mentioned would correspond to that bulk consisting merely of the specific dreaming quality. Maybe this interpretation of the dream-gaps is no more than an analogy ; it might be, however, even more. Yet, it illustrates aptly the incongruence between the interpretable and the original, genuine total dreaming-content.

(19) In dream-interpretation one cannot have a guarantee that one is in every case on the right track ; this will always remain a field where approximately certain knowledge and artistic feeling must go hand-in-hand. The present writer, from the very start of his being an analyist, only with reluctance has used the appellation " dream-interpretation ", for it is too pretentious ; one should rather speak simply of the " *utilisation of dreams in psychotherapy* ". We do not know really *what is* the true and full content of the dreams. When we interpret we try only to arrive at certain conclusions with regard to the various deep mental mechanisms, and to find out certain relations between the dream and the conscious thoughts and sentiments of the dreamer. It depends very much on one's own mental make-up, *how one apperceives*, in the capacity of psychotherapist, the reported dream and association-material. Each of us will be likely to " sense " selectively and mostly those aspects and elements amongst the abundance of the dream-content towards which there exists in his own psyche a preferentially focussed attitude. (We may speak of sub-

---

[1] Cf. p. 5.

conscious attention.) Thus, the present writer has always " perceived psychically " the organic processes of his patients, at the time when he practised as a physician ; he experiences in the same "mental" fashion the physiological events in himself. This colours his conceptions on the dream-phenomena quite obviously, as the critical reader, acquainted with this field, will have noticed. However, we do not run any considerable risk in practical psychotherapy by this selective, individual bias of our mind. For, even though we have regard to only *one* aspect, the subconscious of our patient does not cease to be a *whole*, does not cease to experience its various complexes as a coherent unity ; and, consequently, it reacts in its totality. even though the psychotherapist may have attacked directly only *one* individual aspect. This is most fortunate ; otherwise, the existence of the various contemporary psychotherapeutic schools would be rather a curse to mankind. In fact, these differences in viewpoint have given much stimulation, have cleared up many obscurities and have enriched our knowledge to a considerable extent. This fortunate fact, surely, compensates for the occasionally unpleasant impression which the biased party-spirit of psychologically experienced physicians, and more even that of some lay-analysts,[1] on certain occasions creates. Unfortunately, the fundamental character-traits of an individual and certain, more general, aggressive tendencies, are not considerably changed when one becomes a psychotherapist ; although one might suppose that the liking for psychology would exclude *eo ipso* a tendency towards too conspicuous subjectivism and autism. Unfortunately, this does not seem to be entirely factual. Stekel mentions, in writing the early history of the psychoanalytical movement, a remark of the great Freud, made in an appropriate moment : Psychoanalysis seems to stimulate the worst instincts of man (I quote from memory). It has similarly to be pointed out that a neurotic mental structure—if accompanied by scientific inclination—leads

---

[1] Though I subscribe to the view that the psychotherapist should possess a general medical and psychiatrical-neurological proficiency, I readily admit that there were and are several skilful and even *brilliant* lay-analysts and non-medical psychological authors who contributed much to our field of science. Yet the development of medical psychology aims, obviously, towards the " psychosomatic " unity, even in its theoretical foundation, and it is not fully possible, without thorough knowledge of physiology and pathology, to do justice to the phenomena dealt with in research. Nevertheless, it would be a great loss to exclude from our collaborators anyone who is talented, but owing to circumstances, or even from disinclination, could not comply with the desirable conditions.

some individuals towards psychology. There is no justification for blaming those people for their higher ambitions; yet the fact has to be borne in mind because of some, at first not easily understandable, rare incidents in the *past* literature and life of the psychological societies on the continent.

I should like to admit that, on the other hand, it is not always therapeutically advantageous if the patient feels the absolute objectivity and high-mindedness of his doctor. For our patients are no saints either. They feel it appropriate that the therapist should be just, kind and strong towards them; but co-consciously they also like to see in him a fellow-human-being, who possesses human faults similar to their own, or has, at least, the potential inclination to such "trespasses". I know that some individuals, as patients, cannot bear to think that their analyst is too idealistic in his life; it annoys them and depresses them. Such "allergies" can sometimes be eliminated during the course of the treatment, but not always and not entirely. Thus, from the practical point of view, we can *not* deplore the all-too-human failings of analysts. It would be, of course, better if things were altogether different. But, like the physician in general so the psychotherapist, too, is only a member of the human species; it is still probable that the number of objective, painstaking, healthy personalities *is* somewhat larger among psychotherapists than among the average. Psychological knowledge enhances one's qualities; but nothing that is super-human ought to be demanded of us. We affirm life, i.e., work, duty, pleasure and the satisfaction ensuing from both sources; and in propagating *this* end associated with an optimistic outlook, we are fundamentally suitable to be psychotherapists.

(20) I believe that every "non-dogmatic" dream-analyst, without exception, feels how painful the marked subjectivity of our dream-interpretations is. When considering that the interpretation of any dream, which shows a certain degree of disguising transformation of its latent content, will be rather different, according to the analyst who undertakes it, then one feels a certain "shame for science". This state of affairs must necessarily make the uninitiated very doubtful of the validity of any dream-interpretation. I should expect the greatest similarity between the interpretations of two Adler-followers; no startling differences might be expected in the interpretations of two Freudians, since they would be likely

to emphasise those aspects of the dream which pointed to the
Œdipus—and castration—complexes. Even there, I am not
at all sure about the complete congruity of the various individual interpretations. The greatest differences are usually
observed in the interpretations of the various " free-lance ",
undogmatic analysts, including the followers of Stekel. And
yet, the study of the literature would show that this group in
particular has usually been able to support the essence of their
interpretations by reference to corresponding factual memories,
i.e., to the disclosure of historical material, both of the infantile
and recent periods. I may point to the well written book by
Gutheil, *The Language of Dreams*, which appeared in America
in 1939, and which contains very convincing interpretations.
I knew the author in Vienna—we belonged to Stekel's circle—
as a very successful therapist who, in general, based his treatment on "active dream-interpretation" ; his practical achieve-
ments definitely strengthen his claims for his special interpretations. I myself, several years ago, began a book on this subject ;
having finished the first part I delayed publication because
I could *not* bring out quite convincingly (not even for myself)
the theoretical reasons for the various interpretations. Unfortunately, I lost a great bulk of the notes through the unfavourable circumstances of the present times. These notes dealt
with the various groups of neurosis, i.e., potency-disturbances,
phobias, sleeplessness, compulsion and obsessive neuroses,
dreams in training analysis, etc. ; thus the second part of this
" Special Dream-Interpretation " has to be built up anew.

However, as pointed out, as scientists we cannot simply
ignore this marked difference in the various dream-interpretations. Fortunately, this does not endanger the cause
of practical psychotherapy. In the long, passive analytical
technique, often matters are smoothed out automatically
through the method *per se*, i.e., the time and transference
factors. In the more active form of analytical treatment it
seems sufficient to work on certain aspects of the case ; the
psyche reacts as a whole, and so definitely makes up for what
has perhaps been neglected. Even so it has to be pointed out
that there are patients who go from analyst to analyst till one
day some therapist succeeds in unriddling and interpreting
intuitively a particular dream, by virtue of a certain " affinity ",
a gift in that special direction, and so effects the cure of the
illness. I know that authors have written articles, and even

books, on certain interesting cases ; yet the patient was actually cured only later by a psychologist who was possibly quite young, but, not being limited by certain learned presumptions, he was in the position to guess and to disclose a certain simple historical event. I admit that I should not advise anyone whose natural gifts do not lie in this direction, to venture this "active type" of psychoanalytical treatment without a good training in it. It seems also that a great number of patients who have come for treatment in the last decade, are different from those in earlier periods ; their illness consists more in character difficulties and compulsion symptoms and less frequently in "monosymptoms" of the hysterical and phobic variety. All these people mostly need a different and a rather longer—shall we say Freudian—type of technique. But even in such cases the skilful application of an "intuitive guess" might succeed in persuading a patient, who is about "to fly from insight", to continue treatment. This is then to his own advantage, as well as to the greater glory of the analyst, who will thus be maligned by one person less. (It is sufficiently known that many of those who are "on principle" opponents of psychotherapy, are "resistance-patients", or patients who have been made shy by incautious statements and too hasty interpretations.)

(21) However conditions may be to-day, I believe that the science of dream-interpretation is certainly still *capable of development*. The author has yet to come who will write the "perfect" Dream Book, a work which will give adequate expression to the present state of our factual or probable knowledge. There will be especial need for collecting all the material and results concerning the *different types of dreamers*.[1] By establishing in an early period of the analysis the fundamental character of dreaming of the individual, much useless effort can be avoided, by recognising which recurrent features of the dream series reflect, for instance, a paranoid attitude in general, and which other motifs presumably express complexes, fit for analytical solution.[2] In view of the very great discrepancies mentioned, it is perhaps best at present *not* to claim exclusive validity for any type of interpretation. I am often ashamed of being an analyst when educated, critical

---

[1] Cf. also pp. 21-2, 108, 143, 146, 218, 231.
[2] Cf. "The Question of Prognosis in Psychoanalysis as Indicated by the Dreams."

outsiders, point ironically to the considerable differences of view points in the art of dream-interpretation. They are, of course, by no means always right in this criticism.

Let me emphasise again ; the Freudian conceptions will, as far as I can see, remain as a scaffolding ; parts of them will even be used in their entirety. But the future science of dream-interpretation, as well as that of psychoanalysis in general, will surely be different from the original, classical concept of 20 or 30 years ago.

Many readers will reproach me with being subjective. Indeed, I admit that I have not succeeded in eradicating the rather subjective note from this book. However, I believe that in my presentation of the results reached by others, I have striven always for the greatest possible objectivity. As far as I am consciously aware, I have tried to avoid *mere* polemics, attacks, criticism. This book will prove most useful for young colleagues who have *not yet* adopted definitely one particular aspect and conception on the topic, provided that they are not under the personal " transference-influence " of a strong and dogmatic personality. I myself was for many years under the sole influence of Stekel, although he always stressed my relative independence. But at that time this extended only to a few new ideas. I achieved true independence only later, in the course of years and with greater practical experience. I can now safely say that the conceptions of Freud, Adler and Jung, and the discoveries of Stekel, are by no means in true contrast to each other ; rather complementary. The objective dream investigator and author of the future, in his remoteness from all personal and subjective party-experience, will easily show this. They differ greatly, however, in their usefulness for practical psychotherapy, and perhaps for the treatment of different types of patients.

From the theoretical point of view it is hardly possible, for instance, to see in the anxiety-dreams, and also in the post-traumatic dream experiences (in which the reproduction of a previous accident re-appears at intervals), any suitable counter-argument against the infantile, wishfulfilling energetic root of dreaming, as postulated by Freud. Pathological conditions change and disguise the basic mechanisms throughout the whole field of physiological happening. In a patient with a gastric ulcer the normal or even subnormal quantities of acid-secretion (normal and desirable from the view point of digestion) might provoke pains. Though, as mentioned in Chap. VI, we do *not* find proof and cogent reasons for *this* dream-theory, we must admit that there is no definite way of disproving it. Similarly, the daring, and apparently arbitrary, interpretations of Stekel are lacking chiefly in systematic presentation of their psychological foundation. Perhaps the results obtained by our research and suggestions might facilitate the understanding of these interpretations.

(22) Psychoanalysts not belonging to the closer circle of Jung, find only very rarely his archetypes in the dreams of their patients. It is obvious that the interpretation, and even the approximately right interpretation of different dream figures is feasible without relating them to certain explicit figures of ancient mythology. In fact, those legends and tales only give expression to general human motives known also to present-day man. The deep knowledge of life, of the emotional tendencies of man, of the various family and social constellations facing the individual, is a rich enough source for recognising that content behind the dream material which is being looked for, for therapeutic purposes. However, the acquaintance with the popular children's stories and with the current religious traditions will often enable us to throw the light of understanding upon some obscure dream-images. The figure of " an old woman ", for instance, so frequently constituting a motif of the dreams, without having bearing on a special female person, might be easily understood, if one bears in mind the innumerable stories told to children by naïve grown-ups in which the old woman represents some uncanny secret, or deep wisdom, some warning, etc. One of my patients suffering from agoraphobia, in consequence of a series of traumatic events centred around the married life of the parents, dreamt :

> **103.** I am able to work. I am very busy, but at lunchtime I find myself in a house where all the rooms but one are without light. An old woman comes slowly downstairs and I watch her entering this one bright room.

It would have been easy to interpret the old woman as the mother whose ethical behaviour appeared to the daughter not quite right ; but this " discovery " would not have meant anything new to the patient. I preferred explaining to her that the dream figure represents probably some kind of traditional wisdom she believes in, and which is for her the only enlightening hope (the old woman enters the only bright room, all the others are dark . . .) ; she would be able to recover if only she knew certainly that she will finish life as a respectable, reputable mother and wife. This is the only thing on which she is able to focus her attention in the present, and this one-sidedly concentrated energy expenditure is probably the ultimate source of her agoraphobia.

(23) *I* have *not* treated a very large number of patients ; but I have seen, examined and interpreted, more or less correctly, a considerably large number of dreams. As far as I attained therapeutic results, they were based throughout on dream-interpretations. I regard it as justified, therefore, to publish later my book on special dream-interpretation. I believe one should primarily cite dream-examples from successfully treated cases ; there we have at least a certain degree of guarantee that the dream was not entirely misinterpreted. Perhaps more important to emphasise is the fact that we, psychologically trained physicians enjoy a certain advantage over all our fellow-humans, inasmuch as the " experienced " knowledge of psychic mechanisms, the deeper insight into the colourful, apparently irregular, but really not lawless, activities of the psyche, constitute a valuable and attractive possession. The greatest part of such a joy ensuing from this possession is, so I think, due to our familiarity with the world of dreams. The patient who comes to us for treatment, who unfolds for us his inner life, and gives away the world of his dreams, is at the same time our benefactor ; we certainly owe a debt of gratitude for this gift which our fellow-men so freely grant us. I believe we can express this gratitude, partly by endeavouring to be " personalities ", i.e., individuals who at least more than the average, *try* to remain above the daily struggle and collision of petty interests and forces. The sufferer is happy to subordinate himself to one who stands mentally on a higher plane. He will never be able to overcome entirely the feeling of shame and resistance which will be his, if he believes himself forced, by his malady, to open the secret recesses of his soul to one without honour and dignity. I hope the reader will, with some understanding for my motives, forgive the closing of a book, devoted to the spreading of scientific experience, with a moralistic consideration. But I have often preached also to myself, what I have

R*

written here. During my professional career I have often given lectures to medical men and to laymen on questions of medical and social aspects of psychology. I believe I have never conveyed the impression that there are "right" or "wrong" schools. It does not bring honour to our profession if the outer world knows too much of our (at the moment inevitable) differences; nor is this in the interests of our fellow-men. The normal, and even more the neurotic, unbalanced human being is always prone to take sides, to take part in fights, in resistance and attack; it even happens at times that patients refuse to go to a psychotherapist because he does or does not belong to a certain school. Before I was myself established I tried to recommend a friend of mine to some patients of the clinic, but, unfortunately, he was *not* a member of a school, fashionable at that time in Prague. What interest does all this serve? I always look askance at psychological literature which is destined for educated laymen; it is often so very partial, so very prone to offer a new dogma to people who are frequently suffering from a *repression of their religious needs*—a substitute dogma which they then proceed to defend viciously. I know that most psychologists have, too, the human need to possess a "favourite philosophical belief", and feel an irresistible impulse to gain for it, as for their scientific convictions, the support of numerous followers. It is fundamentally a similar need which drives ethical writers and religious leaders to spread the truth and to augment the number of their disciples. But I believe that in doing so we risk too much that is valuable—the honour of our profession and also therapeutic success. Psychology nowadays is not only Weltanschauung, a way of looking upon life, but a means of therapy.

I said I was not going to polemicise, and yet I am doing just that. I am not, however, arguing against different trends and scientific views, only against regrettable, though very general, human peculiarities, in so far as they threaten to "overshadow" the beautiful field of our psychoanalytical activity. Perhaps, one is no more justified in withholding his experiences and suggestions regarding this "technical" and "social" aspect of psychotherapy from one's younger colleagues than in withholding one's scientific views proper. I am writing these closing lines at a time when the individual is hardly in a position to predict his future in any way. I am saying this to stress that it is not pure conceit and presumption which induces me to give such advice. And, moreover, *I have a genuine respect for all seekers after truth, particularly for all those who endeavour to further human happiness. The physician in general, and the psychotherapist in particular, belong quite definitely to the group of these seekers and benefactors. I, therefore, dedicate this small book of mine in a deeply felt friendship to all my colleagues, and also to all those scientists in other fields who have a genuine interest in medical psychology.*

REFERENCES

ADLER, A. *Der Nervöse Character*, 1912. (*The Neurotic Constitution*. Translated by Gluck and Lind. London (Kegan Paul), 1917.)

BETLHEIM AND HARTMANN. *Über Fehlleistungen des Gedächtnisses in der Korsakoffschen Psychose* (Errors of Memory in Korsakoff-psychosis), *Arch. f. Psych.* 72, 1942.

BJERRE, P. *Das Träumen als Heilungsweg der Seele*. (Dreaming as a Means of Healing the Soul.) Rasher Verlag, Zürich 1936.

ELLIS, H. *The World of Dreams*. London (Constable), 1926.

FECHNER, G. T., quoted by Freud.

FEDERN, P. "Über zwei typische Traumsensationen." (Two Typical Dream-sensations.) *Jahrbuch der Psychan*. VI, and in Freud's *Traumdeutung*, Ch. VI.

FREUD, S. *Die Traumdeutung*, 6th Edition, 1921. (*The Interpretation of Dreams*. Translated from the 8th edition by A. A. Brill. London (Allen & Unwin), 1932.)

—— *Vorlesungen*, 1922. (*Introductory Lectures on Psycho-Analysis*. Translated by J. Riviere. London (Allen & Unwin), 1940)

—— *Neue Folge von Vorlesungen*, 1932. (*New Introductory Lectures on Psycho-Analysis*. Translated by W. J. H. Sprott. London (Hogarth Press), 1933).

—— *Der Traum* 1921. (*On Dreams*. Translated by M. Eder.) London (Heinemann).

GUTHEIL, E. A. *The Language of the Dream*. New York (The Macmillan Co.), 1939.

JONES, E. *Papers on Psycho-Analysis*. (Contains a paper on the Theory of Symbolism.) London (Balliere, Tindall and Cox), 1923.

JUNG, C. G. *Wandlungen und Symbole der Libido* (*Psychology of the Unconscious*. Translated by B. J. Hinkle. London (Kegan Paul), 1922.)

—— *Modern Man in Search of a Soul*. (Contains a lecture on Dreams.) Translated by W. S. Dell and C. F. Baynes. London (Kegan Paul), 1933.

KIMMINS, C. W. *Children's Dreams*. London (Allen & Unwin), 1931.

LOWY, S. " Die intuitive Traumdeutung in der Psychotherapie " (Intuitive Dream-Interpretation in Psychotherapy), in *Bericht des Allg. Ärzt. Kongresses für Psychotherapie*. Verl. Hirzel, Leipzig, 1930.

—— " Die verschiedenen Träume derselben Nacht " (The Various Dreams of the Same Night), *Bericht des Allg. Ärzt. Kongresses für Psychotherapie*. Verl. Hirzel, Leipzig, 1931.

—— " Wiederstandsträume " (Resistance-Dreams), *Fortschritte der Sexualwissenschaft und Psychoanalyse*, Band IV. Verl. Deuticke, Wien.

—— " Eigentümlichkeiten des Behandlungsträume, und Probleme des Behandlungsträume " (Peculiarities and Problems of Dreams during Treatment). *Five articles*, in *Psychoanal. Praxis*, 1931, 1932, 1933. Verl. Hirzel, Leipzig.

248 REFERENCES

LOWY, S. " Zur Frage der Prognosestellung in der Psychoanalyse " (The Question of Prognosis in Psychoanalysis as Indicated by the Dreams) ; *Psychoanal. Praxis*, 4, 1932.

—— " Bestätigung des intuitiven Deutung " (Confirmation of Intuitive Interpretation), in *Psychotherap. Praxis*, 1934. Verl. der Psych. Prax. Wien.

—— " Zum Problem der Tagesreste " (Contribution to the Problem of Day-residues), *Zentrbl. für Psychotherapie*, Bnd. IV. H.1. Verl. Hirzel, Leipzig.

—— " Gedanken zur Psychotherapie paranoider Zustände " (Psychotherapy of Paranoid Conditions), *Psychoanal. Praxis*, 1932. Verl. Hirzel, Leipzig.

—— " Psychotherapie einer paranoiden Psychose " (Psychotherapy of a Case of Paranoid Psychosis). In *Psychother. Praxis*, 1936.

—— " Die biologische Stellung des Traumes " (Biological Status of the Dream), *Nederlandsch Tijdschrift voor Psychologie*, VI, 1938.

MAURY, A. *Le Somneil et les Rêves*, 1878. Quoted by Freud.

NICOLL, M. *Dream Psychology*. Oxford Univ. Press, 1920.

PIERCE, F. *Dreams and Personality*. New York (Appleton), 1931.

PÖTZL, O. " Experimentell erregte Traumbilder," etc. (Experimental Dreams), *Ztschrft. f. ges. Neurol. u. Psychiatr.*, 37, 1917.

RANK, O. " Die Symbolschichtung im Wecktraum " (The Symbol-layers in Awakening-Dreams). *Jahrb. Psy.*, An. IV.

—— *Psychoanalytische Beiträge zur Mythenforschung* (Psychoanalytical Contributions to Mythological Research).

SANTE DE SANCTIS. *Psychologie des Traumes* (Psychology of Dreams), in : *Handbuch der Vergl. Psychologie*, Vol. III. Verl. Reinhardt, München, 1922.

SCHERNER, K. A. *Das Leben des Traumes* (The Dream-Life) 1861. Quoted by Freud.

SCHILDER, P. *Entwurf zu einer Psychiatrie auf Psychoanalytischer Grundlage* (Sketch of a Psycho-analytical Presentation of Psychiatry), Internat. Psychoanal. Verlag, Wien, und Zürich, 1925.

SCHRÖTTER, K. " Experimentelle Träume " (Experimental Dreams.) *Zentrbl. Psy.*, An. II. Quoted by Silberer.

SCHULTZ, I. H. *Das autogene Training* (The Autogene Training), Verl. Thieme, Leipzig, 1932.

SILBERER, H. *Der Traum* (The Dream). F. Enke, Stuttgart, 1919.

STEKEL, W. *Die Sprache des Traumes* (The Language of Dreams.) Verl. Bergmann, München, 1922.

—— *Fortschritte der Traumdeutung* (Advances in Dream-Interpretation.) Verlag. f. Med., Weidmann, Wien, Bern, 1935. Engl. Translation by E. Paul awaits publication.

—— *Störungen des Trieb und Affectlebens* (Disorders of Instinctual and Emotional Life). 10 Volumes. Urban & Schwarzenberg, Wien, 1920–1928. Six volumes are translated into English.

VOLD, J. M. *Über den Traum* (The Dream), 1910 and 1912. Quoted by Freud.

INDEX

Cases